Technical Operating Specifications for Zhuang
Medicine Therapies and Their Applications

壮医适宜技术操作
规范与应用

（中英文版）

主 编　罗艺徽　翟 阳

Editor-in-Chief　Luo Yihui Zhai Yang

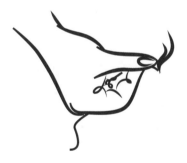

广西科学技术出版社

Guangxi Science & Technology Publishing House

图书在版编目（CIP）数据

壮医适宜技术操作规范与应用：汉文、英文 / 罗艺徽，
翟阳主编. —南宁：广西科学技术出版社，2022.12
ISBN 978-7-5551-1871-8

Ⅰ.①壮… Ⅱ.①罗… ②翟… Ⅲ.①壮医—技术操
作规程—汉、英 Ⅳ.①R291.8-65

中国版本图书馆CIP数据核字（2022）第209109号

ZHUANGYI SHIYI JISHU CAOZUO GUIFAN YU YINGYONG

壮医适宜技术操作规范与应用（中英文版）

主编　罗艺徽　翟　阳

责任编辑：黎志海　吴桐林　　　　　装帧设计：梁　良
责任校对：吴书丽　　　　　　　　　责任印制：韦文印

出　版　人：卢培钊　　　　　　　　出版发行：广西科学技术出版社
社　　　址：广西南宁市东葛路66号　邮政编码：530023
网　　　址：http://www.gxkjs.com

经　　　销：全国各地新华书店
印　　　刷：广西昭泰子隆彩印有限责任公司
开　　　本：787 mm×1092 mm　1/16
字　　　数：262千字　　　　　　　　印　　　张：15.5
版　　　次：2022年12月第1版　　　　印　　　次：2022年12月第1次印刷
书　　　号：ISBN 978-7-5551-1871-8
定　　　价：198.00元

编委会名单

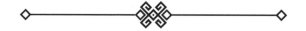

主　编：罗艺徽　翟　阳

副主编：郑光珊　蒋桂江　杨　鹏

编　委：岳桂华　黄国东　李凤珍　王　强　潘明甫

　　　　陈　莹　钟丽雁　蒋咏玲　王成龙　马　艳

　　　　龙朝阳　罗远带　贺诗寓　徐卓妮　覃　信

　　　　苟　尧

主　审：黄汉儒

翻　译：黄登娴 @ 语言桥

资助项目：1. 广西科技基地和人才专项（桂科 AD18281094）

　　　　　2. 2022 年中医药国际交流与合作项目

List of Editorial Board Members

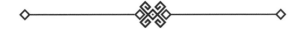

Funded Projects: 1. Guangxi Science and Technology Base and Talents Project
(Guike AD18281094)

2. 2022 TCM International Exchange and Cooperation Project

目　录
Contents

第一章　壮医药物竹罐疗法
Chapter 1　Zhuang Medicine Bamboo Cupping Therapy

第二章　壮医药线点灸疗法
Chapter 2　Zhuang Medicine Medicated Thread Moxibustion

第三章　壮医脐环穴针刺疗法
Chapter 3　Acupuncture at the Umbilical Ring Point in Zhuang Medicine

第四章　壮医药浴疗法
Chapter 4　Zhuang Medicine Medicated Bath Therapy

第一章 壮医药物竹罐疗法
Chapter 1 Zhuang Medicine Bamboo Cupping Therapy

一、疗法概况
I Introduction

壮医药物竹罐疗法是在壮医理论指导下，用煮沸的壮药液加热特制的竹罐，再将竹罐趁热吸拔于患者治疗部位上，利用其负压吸力、药物及温热共同起效，以达防病治病目的的一种独特壮医外治疗法。可以配合壮医刺血疗法、壮医药熨疗法以增加疗效。

The Zhuang medicine (ZM) bamboo cupping therapy, a distinctive external therapeutic method in accordance with the ZM theories, involves putting a bamboo cup onto applied areas after being boiled in a herbal decoction such that the negative fluid pressure of air, herbal medicinals and heat can take synergistic effect to prevent and treat diseases. It can also be combined with Zhuang medical therapies of bloodletting pricking and hot ironing to increase treatment efficacy.

本法流传于广西壮族聚居地区，历史悠久。其使用广西盛产的金竹制作成的竹罐和道地壮药，适应病证范围广，可用于治疗临床各科疾病，主要用于发旺（风湿病）关节痛、核嘎尹（腰腿痛）、颈椎病、肩背酸痛等痛症，痧病，甫裆呷（半身不遂），麻抹（麻木），骨折愈后瘀积等。尤其是对发旺（风湿病）关节痛，消肿止痛疗效显著。安全无毒副作用。

Widely used in the settlements of the Zhuang nationality in Guangxi, this therapy is an ancient treatment method in which cups made of Jinzhu (*Phyllostachys sulphurea*) native to Guangxi and authentic Zhuang medicine is applied to treat a wide range of diseases such as rheumatic diseases ("Fawang" in ZM), lumbago and leg pain ("Hegayin" in ZM), cervical spondylosis, shoulder and back pain, filthy-attack eruptive disease, hemiplegia ("Bengdangga" in ZM), numbness ("Mamo" in ZM) and blood stasis after fracture recovery. Among those diseases, in particular, this therapy has apparent effectiveness in relieving joint swelling and pain caused by rheumatism. It is safe and free from toxic and side effect.

（一）发展历史

1 History of the ZM bamboo cupping therapy

壮医药物竹罐疗法是壮族先民在与疾病进行长期斗争的过程中积累下来的宝贵经验，是壮族特色传统医疗技法之一，在广西壮族聚居地区流传历史悠久，主要流传于壮族聚居的德保县、靖西市、乐业县等地。其中，乐业县的老壮医岑利族家族世代行医，擅长骨科疾病及发旺（风湿病）的治疗，因为当地群众解除病痛而远近闻名。他们主要运用壮医药物竹罐疗法治疗发旺（风湿病）关节痛、核嘎尹（腰腿痛）、肩背酸痛、麻抹（麻木）、甭裆呷（半身不遂）、林得叮相（跌打损伤）、巧尹（头痛）、骨折愈后瘀积等，受到广大民众的赞赏和欢迎。当地民间流传着这样一句俗语："扎针拔罐子，病好大半子。"但是，由于缺乏文字记载，壮医药物竹罐疗法只通过口耳相传的方式流传下来。自 1985 年广西民族医药研究所（现广西民族医药研究院）成立后，黄汉儒所长带领科研人员对广西少数民族医药进行发掘整理，壮医药物竹罐疗法正是被发掘整理出来的壮医特色疗法之一。通过临床验证其疗效和安全性，证明该疗法疗效显著、安全、无毒副作用，因此，在临床上应用于治疗痧病、各种原因引起的核嘎尹（腰腿痛）、颈椎病、肩背酸痛、麻抹（麻木）、甭裆呷（半身不遂）、肌肤痹冷疼痛不适、骨折愈后瘀积、林得叮相（跌打损伤）、巧尹（头痛）等。广西民族医药研究院李凤珍主任医师临床应用其治疗风湿病等，并进行技术规范与推广应用，其提出的壮医药物竹罐疗法治疗膝骨关节炎的技术被列为广西基层常见病多发病壮医适宜技术，在广西区内外推广应用，成效显著。壮医药物竹罐疗法 2013 年入选南宁市非物质文化遗产项目，2015 年入选广西壮族自治区非物质文化遗产项目，代表性传承人为李凤珍。多年来，李凤珍一直在临床应用与研究中传承并推广应用壮医药物竹罐疗法。

The ZM bamboo cupping therapy represents valuable experience accumulated by the ancestors of the Zhuang nationality in their long-term struggle with diseases.

This distinctive ancient therapeutic technique is widely used in the settlements of the Zhuang nationality in Guangxi, including the counties of Debao, Jingxi and Leye. Cen Lizu from Leye County, whose family has practiced ZM for several generations, excels at curing orthopedic diseases and rheumatic diseases ("Fawang" in ZM), winning a reputation. They applied the therapy to treat diseases such as rheumatic arthralgia ("Fawang" in ZM), lumbago and leg pain ("Hegayin" in ZM), shoulder and back pain, numbness ("Mamo" in ZM), hemiplegia ("Bengdangga" in ZM), injury from knocks and falls ("Lindedingxiang" in ZM), headache ("Qiaoyin" in ZM) and blood stasis after fracture recovery. There is a folk saying that "needling and cupping enable people to recover from diseases more quickly". Therefore, the ZM bamboo cupping therapy is popular in the locality, but it had been imparted from one generation to another by word of mouth until Huang Hanru, the director of Guangxi Institute of Minority Medicine established in 1985, and his team recorded it in written form. As one of distinctive Zhuang medical therapies collated by the team, the ZM bamboo cupping therapy has passed the clinical trial process, proving to be effective, safe and free from toxic and side effects. This approved therapy has been used to effectively treat many diseases, including filthy-attack eruptive disease, lumbago and leg pain ("Hegayin" in ZM), cervical spondylosis, shoulder and back pain, numbness ("Mamo" in ZM), hemiplegia ("Bengdangga" in ZM), cold and pain in muscles, blood stasis after fracture recovery, injury from knocks and falls ("Lindedingxiang" in ZM) and headache ("Qiaoyin" in ZM). Li Fengzhen, a chief physician at Guangxi Institute of Minority Medicine, applies the ZM bamboo cupping therapy to mainly treat the rheumatic disease while formulating its technical specifications and promoting its applications. The technique described in her program *The Zhuang Medicine Bamboo Cupping Therapy in the treatment of knee osteoarthritis* is designated as an appropriate technique to treat common diseases in the settlements of the Zhuang nationality in Guangxi. It has also been introduced to other places and widely applied. The ZM bamboo cupping therapy was inscribed on the Representative List of Intangible Cultural Heritage of Humanity at Nanning City level in 2013 and at Guangxi Zhuang Autonomous Region level in 2015, and at the same time, Li Fengzhen was designated as the representative inheritor since she had devoted herself to the application of this therapy and its popularization during her clinical treatment and research.

（二）治疗机理
2　Treatment mechanism

壮医药物竹罐疗法的治疗机理是用煮沸的壮药液加热特制的竹罐，再将竹罐趁热吸拔于患者治疗部位的皮肤上，以疏通龙路、火路气机，达到祛风除湿、活血舒筋、散寒止痛、拔毒消肿等治疗效果。从现代医学的观点来看，在拔罐时，除负压吸拔的良性刺激外，拔罐部位吸收药气，加上温热作用，可扩张局部血管，加速血液循环，改善血液流变学状态，调节神经系统、免疫系统功能，清除体内代谢终产物，从而达到治疗的目的。

The ZM bamboo cupping therapy involves putting a bamboo cup onto applied areas, after being boiled in a herbal decoction. It is used to unblock the dragon and fire channels to dispel wind, remove dampness, activate blood to relax tendons, dissipate cold, relieve pain and draw out toxins to eliminate swelling. From a perspective of modern medicine, when cups are put on the skin, the negative fluid pressure of air, herbal medicinals and heat work together to accelerate blood circulation by dilating regional blood vessels to improve blood flow, and thereby regulate the function of the nervous system and immune system and eliminate metabolic end products.

（三）主要功效
3　Main efficacy

壮医药物竹罐疗法具有祛风除湿，活血舒筋，散寒止痛，拔毒消肿，疏通龙路、火路气机等功效。

The ZM bamboo cupping therapy can be applied to dispel wind, remove dampness, activate blood to relax tendons, dissipate cold, relieve pain, draw out toxins to eliminate swelling and unblock the dragon and fire channels.

二、技法特色

Ⅱ　Characteristics of the therapy

（一）理论特色

1　Theoretical features

根据壮医"毒虚致病"理论，壮医认为，毒侵袭人体，使三道两路不通、气血运行不畅、阴阳不能平衡、三气不能同步而致病。壮医药物竹罐疗法通过局部吸拔刺激，加上药力、热力等作用，疏通龙路、火路，促进气血运行，调节阴阳平衡，祛除邪毒，使恶血得去，疾病得除，机体自安。因此，其理论特色主要是祛毒、调和气血、平衡阴阳、祛除疾病。

According to the theory of "diseases resulting from toxin and deficiency" in ZM, toxin is one of the main factors causing diseases since the three passages and two channels[*] will be blocked when it enters the human body, which results in stagnation of qi and blood movement, yin-yang disharmony and the failure of synchronization of the heaven-qi, earth-qi and human-qi. As a result, diseases occur. The ZM bamboo cupping therapy whereby the negative fluid pressure of air, herbal medicinals and heat work together can be used to unblock the dragon and fire channels, promote the circulation of blood and qi, regulate yin and yang, remove pathogenic toxins. When static blood is cleaned up, the disease will be cured and thus the human body remains healthy. Therefore, the theoretical features of this therapy can be summarized as removing toxins, harmonizing qi and blood and balancing yin with yang.

（二）临床特色

2　Clinical features

（1）本疗法集药力、热力、负压于一体，因此具有祛风毒、除湿毒、化瘀毒、散寒毒的作用，尤其祛瘀疗效甚优，消肿痛疗效确切，而且起效快，作用较持久。

---

　　[*] The three passages refer to the water passage, the grain passage and the qi passage; the two channels refer to the dragon channel and the fire channel.

(1) The ZM bamboo cupping therapy enables herbal medicinals, heat and negative fluid pressure of air to take the synergistic effect to dispel wind, remove dampness, dissipate blood stasis and disperse cold. In particular, this therapy has quick-acting efficacy and long-lasting efficacy on removal of blood stasis and elimination of swelling.

（2）本疗法使用的竹罐轻巧，操作灵活，适用于任意大小部位的治疗，尤其适宜较小关节部位的治疗。

(2) The light and small bamboo cups used in this therapy can be placed on any applied areas, especially suitable for small articular surfaces.

（3）适应病证范围广，可用于治疗临床各科疾病，主要用于发旺（风湿病）关节痛、核嘎尹（腰腿痛）、颈椎病、肩背酸痛等痛症，痧病，甭裆呷（半身不遂），麻抹（麻木），骨折愈后瘀积等病证。尤其是对发旺（风湿病）关节疼痛肿胀，消肿止痛疗效显著。

(3) The therapy can be used to treat a wide range of diseases, including rheumatic diseases ("Fawang" in ZM), lumbago and leg pain ("Hegayin" in ZM), cervical spondylosis, shoulder and back pain, filthy-attack eruptive disease, hemiplegia ("Bengdangga" in ZM), numbness ("Mamo" in ZM) and blood stasis after fracture recovery. In particular, this therapy has great efficacy on relief of joint pain and swelling induced by rheumatism ("Fawang" in ZM).

（4）简便验廉、无毒副作用、无污染。

(4) The therapy is of simple and convenient operation, effective and cheap. The materials used are free from toxic and side effect and pollution.

（三）选穴特色
3   Features of acupoints selection

以局部阿是穴为主，再视病变情况取邻近部位的常用穴位。

Normally, Ashi points at the affected area are selected, combined with adjacent acupoints as appropriate.

（1）病变部位取穴。一般根据病变部位局部取阿是穴，如疼痛、压痛、肿胀等部位。

(1) Selection of disease sites. Ashi points at the areas of the disease site, such as painful, tenderness elicited and swollen areas, are selected.

（2）邻近部位取穴。壮医认为，大多数穴位都可以治疗该穴位所在部位及邻近部位的病证。因此，当某一部位病变时，可以在该部位局部或邻近部位取穴。如腰背痛，则取腰背部穴位如腰眼、夹脊；肩周炎则取肩关节前、后、上三面周围穴位。

(2) Selection of adjacent acupoints. In ZM, points in or near the affected area are normally selected for treatment. For example, points on the back and lower back such as Yaoyan (EX-B 7) and Jiaji (EX-B 2) are selected for treatment of lumbago and back pain while points around the anterior, posterior and upper sides of the shoulder joint for scapulohumeral periarthritis.

（3）经验取穴。通过临床积累总结形成一些取穴经验，如痧病取背部、颈部；头痛取背部、颈部、额中、印堂、太阳；腹痛取脐周四穴。

(3) Acupoints selection according to experience. Normally, the selection of Acupoints is based on clinical experience. For example, points on the back and neck are selected for filthy-attack eruptive disease, points on the back and neck and in the middle of the forehead, Yintang (EX-HN 3) and Taiyang (EX-HN 5) for headache, while points around the navel for abdominal pain.

三、操作规范
Ⅲ　Specifications for operation

（一）前期准备
1　Pre-treatment preparation

用物准备。

Prepare the materials for the application of the therapy.

（1）竹罐：10～20个（图1）。

(1) Cups: 10~20 bamboo cups (Fig. 1).

（2）壮药：根据病证选择相应壮药（图2）。

(2) Zhuang herbal medicinals: Select Zhuang medicinals in accordance with the disease (Fig. 2).

（3）其他：电磁炉、不锈钢锅或其他锅具，消毒毛巾，长镊子，一次性注射针头，无菌手套，复合碘皮肤消毒液，医用棉签，无菌纱布，无菌棉球，浴巾。

(3) Other items: An induction cooker or a stainless steel pot or other pots, disinfectant towels, long tweezers, disposable injection needles, sterile gloves, compound iodine disinfectant, medical cotton swabs, sterile gauze, aseptic cotton balls and bath towels.

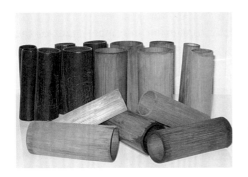

图 1　竹罐

Fig. 1　Bamboo cups

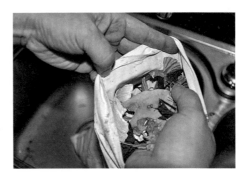

图 2　壮药

Fig. 2　Zhuang herbal medicinals

（二）操作流程

2　Operating procedure

1. 药液准备

2.1　Preparation for herbal decoction

将药物装入布袋，加水浸泡至少30分钟，然后煮沸用于浸煮竹罐（图3）。

Put Zhuang medicinals into a cloth bag and heat the bag with water after leaving it to soak in water for at least 30 minutes. Then, boil bamboo cups in the herbal decoction (Fig. 3).

2. 体位选择

2.2　Patient positioning

根据病情确定体位，常让患者取坐位、卧位，以患者舒适及便于施术者操作为宜，避免用强迫体位。

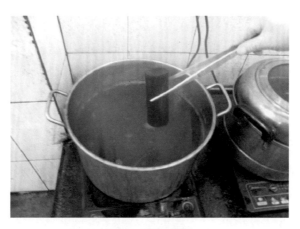

图 3　浸煮竹罐

Fig. 3　Decoct Zhuang medicinals with water and boil bamboo cups in the herbal decoction

The selection of proper patient positioning aims to provide patient comfort and make the treatment site optimally exposed.

（1）仰卧位。吸拔前胸、腹部和上下肢的前侧部位时采用仰卧位。

(1) Supine position. This position is used for placing cups on the anterior side of the chest and extremities, and the abdomen.

（2）俯卧位。吸拔腰背部、下肢后侧部位时采用俯卧位。

(2) Prone position. This position is used for placing cups on the back, lower back and the posterior side of the lower extremities.

（3）侧卧位。适用于周身除接触床的部位外的各个部位。

(3) Lateral position. This position can be used for placing cups on any sides of the body except the one on the bed.

（4）坐位。吸拔颈部、肩部、上肢及膝部时采用坐位。

(4) Sitting position. This position is used for placing cups on the neck, shoulders, upper extremities and knees.

3. 部位选择

2.3　Selection of acupoints

根据病证选取适当治疗部位或穴位（表 1）。一般每次治疗部位 ≤ 4 个。

Normally, no more than 4 acupoints are selected according to medical conditions (Tab. 1).

常选局部阿是穴为主，可配合邻近部位取穴。如腰背痛取阿是穴，可取腰背部穴位如腰眼、夹脊；肩痛取阿是穴，可取肩关节前、后、上三面周围穴位；腰痛取阿是穴，可取肾俞、腰俞、腰阳关、次髎等穴位；腿痛取阿是穴，可取环跳、阴市、伏兔、委中、阳陵泉、绝骨等穴位；上肢痛取阿是穴，可取肩髃、合谷、外关、曲池等穴位；痧症需取胸背部肌肉较丰厚处的穴位，可取太阳、合谷、外关等穴位。

From the perspective of ZM, normally, Ashi points in the affected area are selected as the primary ones while those close to the disease site are taken as the secondary ones for treatment, for example, Ashi points on the back and lower back such as Yaoyan (EX-B 7) and Jiaji (EX-B 2) for lumbago and back pain; Ashi points around the anterior, posterior and upper sides of the shoulder joint for scapulohumeral periarthritis; Ashi points including Shenshu (BL 23), Yaoshu (GV 2), Yaoyangguan (GV 3) and Ciliao (BL 32) for lower back pain; Ashi points including Huantiao (GB 30), Yinshi (ST 33), Futu (ST 32), Weizhong (BL 40), Yanglingquan (GB 34), Juegu (GB 39) for leg pain; Ashi points including Jianyu (LI 15), Hegu (LI 4), Waiguan (TE 5) and Quchi (LI 11) for upper extremity pain and Ashi points on the thick muscle layers of the chest and back for filthy-attack eruptive disease, including Taiyang (EX-HN 5), Hegu (LI 4) and Waiguan (TE 5).

表1 壮医药物竹罐治疗各部位拔罐数

部位	罐数
颈部（包括上背、颈）	≤ 12 罐
背部	≤ 20 罐
腰部	≤ 20 罐
单侧肩关节（包括肩周、肩胛区）	≤ 16 罐
单侧肘关节（包括肘、上臂、前臂）	≤ 10 罐
单侧腕关节（包括腕、手背、前臂）	≤ 6 罐
双侧臀部	≤ 16 罐
单侧膝关节	≤ 10 罐
单侧踝关节	≤ 8 罐
单侧上肢	≤ 12 罐
单侧下肢	≤ 16 罐

Tab. 1　The Number of Bamboo Cups Used for Each Affected Area

Applied area	Number of cups
Neck (the upper back and the neck)	≤ 12
Back	≤ 20
Lumbar region	≤ 20
Shoulder joint (the scapula and periscapular region)	≤ 16 (for each side)
Elbow joint (the elbow, the upper arm and the forearm)	≤ 10 (for each side)
Wrist joint (the wrist, the back of hand and the forearm)	≤ 6 (for each side)
Buttocks	≤ 16
Knee joint	≤ 10 (for each side)
Ankle joint	≤ 8 (for each side)
Upper extremity	≤ 12 (for each side)
Lower extremity	≤ 16 (for each side)

4. 消毒

2.4　Sterilization

洗手，戴口罩、医用帽及一次性无菌手套。

Wash hands and wear masks, medical hats and disposable aseptic gloves.

5. 操作步骤

2.5　The cupping process

（1）患者选择合适的体位，暴露治疗部位。

(1) Positioning. Place the patient in a proper position to make the treatment site exposed.

（2）煮罐。将竹罐投入药液中，煮沸 5 分钟备用。

(2) Cup boiling. Boil the bamboo cups in the boiled herbal decoction for 5 minutes.

（3）第一次拔罐。根据拔罐部位选定大小合适的竹罐，从锅中捞出后甩尽水珠（也可以迅速用折叠的消毒毛巾捂一下罐口，以便吸去药液，降低罐口的温度并保持罐内的热气），迅速扣于选定的部位上，5～10 分钟后取下竹罐（图 4）。

(3) The first cupping. Choose right-sized cups for applied areas, shake them to remove water (or immediately cover the cup rim with a sterilized towel to lower

the temperature of the rim and keep the heat in the cup interior) and place them onto applied areas for 5~10 minutes (Fig. 4).

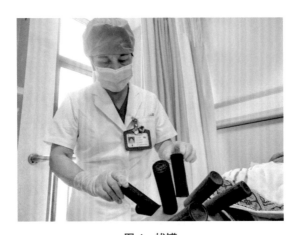

图 4　拔罐
Fig. 4　Cupping

（4）可配合做壮医刺血疗法。根据患者病情及体质情况判断，如果拔罐后罐印部位瘀血较重，可在罐印部位配合做壮医刺血疗法，即常规消毒皮肤，用一次性注射针头在罐印部位皮肤上迅速浅刺（0.1～0.3 cm）1～3针，以局部少量渗血为度。

(4) ZM bloodletting pricking. According to the patient's medical and physical conditions, combine bloodletting pricking with cupping for heavy blood stasis at applied areas. Specifically, after having applied cupping, sterilize the site and prick it quickly with a disposable injection needle. Normally, insert the needle into the skin with a depth of 0.1~0.3 cm 1~3 times so as to remove a small amount of the static blood.

（5）第二次拔罐。另取煮热的竹罐在刺血部位再次拔罐，5～10分钟后取下竹罐，用无菌棉球擦净血迹后常规消毒皮肤。

(5) The second cupping. Place another boiled cups onto the pricked site for 5~10 minutes and remove them. Then, sterilize the site after wiping off the blood stains with aseptic cotton balls.

（6）可配合做壮医药熨疗法。拔罐后用药巾（将消毒毛巾浸于热药液中，捞出拧半干即成）热熨拔罐部位，待温度合适时在拔罐部位热敷5～10分钟。

(6) Zhuang medicine ironing therapy. After removing the cups, press and rub the site with a medical towel (i. e. a sterilized, decoction-saturated towel which is wrung to remove excessive decoction). Then, retain the towel on the site for 5~10 minutes when its temperature is proper.

注：如果为病情较轻或一般，或晕血者，第一次拔罐后接着做壮医药熨疗法即结束；如患者病情较重，且体质壮实、无晕血，第一次拔罐后，拔罐部位瘀血较重者可配合做壮医刺血疗法，第二次拔罐后再做壮医药熨疗法。

Note: For those with mild blood stasis or hemophobia, the treatment ends up with Zhuang medicine ironing therapy after Step (3) is performed; for those with severe blood stasis but with strong constitution and without hemophobia, perform the treatment, following Step (3) ~Step (6).

6. 治疗时间及疗程

2.6　Treatment session and course

拔罐治疗的时间及疗程根据不同的疾病以及病情的轻重和病程的长短而定。一般来说，每次治疗 40 ～ 50 分钟，急性病每日治疗 1 次，慢性病可每 2 ～ 3 日甚至每周治疗 1 次，治疗 5 ～ 7 次为 1 个疗程。

The lengths of a cupping session and course depend on the severity and course of a disease. But typically, a course consists of five to seven sessions of which each lasts about 40~50 minutes. A treatment is performed one time per day for acute diseases while one time every two or three days or per week for chronic diseases.

（三）注意事项

3　Cautions

（1）让患者选择舒适体位。拔罐过程中不可随便移动体位，以免引起患者疼痛或竹罐脱落，同时要避免患者晕罐。

(1) Place the patient in a comfortable position without change during treatment to protect them from experiencing pain and dizziness and prevent the cups from falling off.

（2）选择肌肉丰厚、皮下组织松弛及毛发少的部位为宜，多毛部位则剃毛。

(2) Preferably put the cups on an area with a thick muscle layer, sagging hypodermis or less hair, if the cups have to be placed on a hairy area, the hair must be shaved prior to treatment.

（3）拔罐一般于饭后 2 小时进行，避免患者因过度饥饿而晕罐。

(3) Perform the cupping therapy 2 hours after a meal to protect the patient from experiencing dizziness due to starvation.

（4）扣罐前尽量甩干竹罐上的水珠以免烫伤患者皮肤。

(4) Remove water on the cups as much as possible before putting them on applied areas to avoid skin burns.

（5）取罐时按压罐边使空气进入，即能取下，不能硬拉药罐。

(5) When removing a cup, press the skin along the edge on its rim with fingertips to release the suction. Never pull the cup directly off the skin.

（6）拔罐后如皮肤起水疱，小者可用万花油涂擦，几天后即能自愈；大者用一次性针头挑破，挤干水后涂上万花油即可。

(6) After cupping, for small blisters, gently apply Wanhua oil to blisters which will disappear in several days; for large blisters, pump out the water in them with a disposable needle before applying Wanhua oil.

（7）长期使用糖皮质激素导致皮肤萎缩者留罐时间短，约 5 分钟即可。

(7) For skin atrophy caused by long-term use of corticosteroids, keep the cups on the spot for a short period of time, usually about 5 minutes.

（8）拔罐后宜饮适量温开水，可加少许食盐；注意保暖、避风寒；拔罐部位保持干燥，当天避免接触冷水，以防受寒及感染。

(8) Advise the patient drinking some warm water into which a bit salt can be added, and keep the skin in applied areas warm and dry. Do not expose the skin to cold water to prevent cold and infection.

（9）依照医院感染预防和控制要求，使用过的竹罐、毛巾送消毒供应中心统一消毒。

(9) In accordance with the required infection prevention and control practices in the healthcare setting, collect all used bamboo cups and towels to the disinfection supply center for sterilization.

（10）以下几类人群忌用或慎用：自发性出血或损伤后不易止血者；局部皮肤溃烂者；体质虚弱、极度消瘦、皮肤没有弹性者；脑血管、心血管、肝、肾及造血系统等严重原发性疾病患者；精神病患者；孕妇及婴幼儿。

(10) Warnings: Apply with caution or do not apply the bamboo cupping therapy to those who have spontaneous bleeding or whose bleeding from a wound is hard to stop; who have local skin ulceration; whose constitution is weak with extreme emaciation, and skin is saggy; who have serious primary diseases in organs including cerebral vessels, blood vessels of the heart, the liver, kidney or hematopoietic system; who have mental illnesses; who are pregnant; and who are aged 0~3.

四、常见病证治疗
Ⅳ　Treatment of common diseases

（一）骆芡（骨关节炎）
1　Osteoarthritis ("Luoqian" in ZM)

1. 疾病概述
1.1　General description

骆芡缘于年老体虚，或受伤留瘀，感受邪毒（风毒、寒毒、湿毒等），客于筋骨，阻滞龙路、火路，使天、地、人三气不能同步而致病。相当于中医的骨痹、西医的骨关节炎。

"Luoqian", also known as bone impediment in traditional Chinese medicine (TCM) and osteoarthritis in Western medicine (WM), often occurs in people with weak constitution due to aging or with blood stasis after injury. Under such circumstances, the body tends to be attacked by pathogenic toxins such as wind, cold and dampness. Subsequently, the static blood and toxins stagnate in tendons and bones and then block the dragon and fire channels. The blockage makes the heaven-qi, earth-qi and human-qi unable to be synchronized, leading to the onset of the disease.

骨关节炎是一种关节软骨进行性消失，骨质过度增生，临床出现慢性关节疼痛、僵硬、肿大、畸形及活动受限等症状的常见风湿病。多发于 50 岁以上的中老年人，好发于负重大、活动多的关节。膝是最常累及的关节之一，故膝骨关节炎最为常见，主要临床表现有膝关节疼痛、僵硬、肿大、畸形及活动受限，严重者出现膝内翻或外翻畸形，不能行走，严重影响生活质量。

Osteoarthritis (OA), the most common form of arthritis, is characterized by loss of arthrodial cartilage over time and bone hyperplasia. The clinical manifestations of osteoarthritis include chronic joint pain, stiffness, swelling, bone spurs and loss of flexibility. OA is often found in people aged 50 or over, Weight-bearing and overused joints are most prone to OA, so as one of the most frequently involved joints, knee osteoarthritis is the most widespread disorder. The clinical manifestations are knee pain, stiffness, swelling, bone spurs and loss of flexibility. Severe knee OA can affect the quality of life since it leads to a valgus and varus deformity which results in significant difficulties with walking.

2. 病因病机

1.2　Cause and mechanism of disease

本病多缘于年老体虚，或受伤留瘀，感受邪毒（风毒、寒毒、湿毒等），客于筋骨，阻滞龙路、火路，使天、地、人三气不能同步而致病。

OA often occurs in people with weak constitution due to aging or with blood stasis after injury. Under such circumstances, the body tends to be attacked by pathogenic toxins such as wind, cold and dampness. Subsequently, the static blood and toxins stagnate in tendons and bones and then block the dragon and fire channels. The blockage makes the heaven-qi, earth-qi and human-qi unable to be synchronized, leading to the onset of the disease.

3. 诊查要点

1.3　Essentials for diagnosis

（1）主症。膝、手、足、腰、颈、髋等关节疼痛，甚或肿胀，屈伸不利，活动时关节常有喀喇声或摩擦声，动辄痛甚，重则关节变形，气候变化时加重，反复不愈。

(1) Main symptoms. Pain in the joints of knees, hands, feet, waist, necks and hips, which may be accompanied by swelling, reduced flexion and extension, clicking or grinding noises during movement which worsens pain, joint deformity with

deterioration of OA, aggravation of pain by climate change and recurrence of pain.

（2）兼症。筋骨酸软，乏力，发僵，麻木，畏寒肢冷。

(2) Concurrent symptoms. Aching, weakness, stiffness and numbness in tendons and bones, intolerance of cold and cold extremities.

（3）目诊。勒答上龙脉脉络弯曲、延伸、有瘀点。

(3) Eye examination. The blood vessels of the eyes are curved and stretched, with petechiae.

（4）甲诊。症轻者甲色淡红，症重者甲色或青或紫或苍白，半月痕暴露过少或过多。

(4) Nail examination. The nails of patients with mild OA are light red while those of patients with severe OA are blue, purple or pale, with small or large fingernail lunulae.

（5）本病多见于中老年人，起病隐匿，发病缓慢。

(5) OA most often affects middle-age to elderly people. It begins insidiously with slow progression.

（6）X射线摄影胶片可见关节面软骨下骨质硬化，骨赘形成，关节间隙狭窄；部分可有骨质疏松改变。

(6) Subchondral bone sclerosis on the articular surface, bone hyperplasia and joint space narrowing can be seen on X-ray image. It can also be seen that some bones have a tendency to become weak and brittle.

（7）查类风湿因子、抗环瓜氨酸抗体、血尿酸等有助于鉴别诊断。

(7) The rheumatoid factor (RF) test, anti-citrulline antibody test and uric acid test can help the diagnosis of OA.

4. 辨证论治

1.4　Syndrome differentiation and treatment

（1）治疗原则。祛风除湿，活血舒筋，散寒止痛，拔毒消肿，通龙路、火路气机。

(1) Treatment principles. Dispel wind, remove dampness, activate blood to relax tendons, dissipate cold, relieve pain, draw out toxins to eliminate swelling and move qi in the dragon and fire channels.

（2）适宜证型。适用于阳证、阴证伴有瘀毒者。

(2) Indications. Yang syndrome or yin syndrome with blood stasis.

（3）壮药。选用杜仲藤、海风藤等。

(3) Zhuang herbal medicinals. Duzhongteng (Cortex Parabarii), Haifengteng (Caulis Piperis Kadsurae), etc.

（4）治疗部位或穴位。以局部阿是穴为主，再视关节病变情况取邻近穴位。局部阿是穴主要选取关节疼痛或肿胀的部位（图5）。邻近穴位包括膝关常穴（鹤顶、足三里、阴陵泉、阳陵泉）、肩关常穴（肩髃、肩贞、肩前）、肘关常穴（曲池、肘髎、曲泽）、腕关常穴（阳池、大陵、外关）、掌指关常穴（合谷、中渚、腕骨）、髋关常穴（环跳、髀关、居髎）、踝关常穴（解溪、冲阳、丘墟）、跖趾关常穴（太冲、内庭、足临泣）。

(4) Acupoints selection. Select Ashi points on the affected area as the primary ones and take adjacent points as secondary ones if necessary (Fig. 5). Specifically, select Ashi points on the painful or swollen joint areas and adjacent points, including Heding (EX-LE 2), Zusanli (ST 36), Yinlingquan (SP 9), Yanglingquan (GB 34), Jianyu (LI 15), Jianzhen (SI 9), Jianqian (EX-UE 12), Quchi (LI 11), Zhouliao (LI 12), Quze (PC 3), Yangchi (TE 4), Daling (PC 7), Waiguan (TE 5), Hegu (LI 4), Zhongzhu (TE 3), Wangu (SI 4), Huantiao (GB 30), Biguan (ST 31), Juliao (GB 29), Jiexi (ST 41), Chongyang (ST 42), Qiuxu (GB 40), Taichong (LR 3), Neiting (ST 44) and Zulinqi (GB 41).

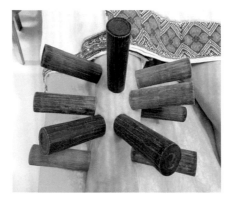

图 5　壮医药物竹罐疗法治疗膝骨关节炎

Fig. 5　Treatment of knee osteoarthritis with the ZM bamboo cupping therapy

（5）具体操作步骤如前述。

(5) The process of treatment for knee OA is the same as that described in Paragraph 2.5 (The cupping process) of Section Ⅲ.

5. 预防调护

1.5　Prevention and care

（1）饮食调理。饮食宜清淡，多食富含胶质和钙的食物。如果身体肥胖，需要适当控制饮食。食疗方可用猪骨黑豆汤、核桃芝麻糊等。

(1) Dietary adjustments. A diet low in fat and salt but high in colloid and calcium is preferable. Calorie-controlled diets are recommended to those who are obese. Recommended dietary supplements are pork bone soup with black beans, walnut sesame paste, etc.

（2）生活起居。劳逸结合，注意保暖，如果身体肥胖，需要减肥。受累关节应避免过度负重，膝关节或髋关节受累患者应避免长久维持站姿、跪姿和蹲姿，可利用手杖、步行器等协助活动。

(2) Daily life. Patients should balance rest and work and keep themselves warm. If they are obese, they should lose weight. Avoid putting additional stress caused by excess weight on weight-bearing joints. Those who have problems with knee or hip joints should avoid a prolonged standing, kneeling or squatting position. Walking aids like a cane or walker can be used for movement.

（3）情志调摄。帮助患者正确认识病情，了解治疗方法、过程及锻炼方法，树立战胜疾病的信心。

(3) Emotional adjustments. Patients should understand OA, the treatment procedure as well as exercises for it, which will help them to establish confidence in curing it.

（4）关节功能锻炼。急性期应减少病变关节过度活动，可卧床休息；症状缓解后，应积极进行锻炼，以关节的非负荷运动及增强肌力和耐力的运动为主，如散步、游泳。针对不同关节的功能障碍选择适宜的康复训练方法，主要是肌力训练和关节活动度训练。

(4) Joint mobility exercises. Patients in the acute stage of OA should less use the affected joints and can opt to rest in bed. When the symptoms of OA are relieved,

they should do regular non-load exercises for increasing strength and endurance of muscles on and around joints, for example, walking and swimming. In terms of movement dysfunction rehabilitation, exercises for different joints may vary but aim to increase muscle strength and joint range of motion.

6. 医案选读

1.6　Selected case readings

【病案一】

［Case 1］

蒋某，女，80 岁，2021 年 1 月 4 日初诊。

Patient: Jiang, an 80-year-old woman; her first visit was on January 4, 2021.

主诉：双膝反复疼痛 10 年，加重 10 个月。

Chief complaint:"I have had recurrent bilateral knee pain in the past ten years, which became worse ten months ago."

现病史：患者 10 年前出现双膝关节疼痛，上下楼梯时明显，伴下蹲、蹲起活动受限。医院诊断为骨关节炎，未系统诊治，症状反复，劳累后加重，休息减轻。10 个月前，双膝关节疼痛明显，行走困难，出现间歇性跛行，跛行距离不定，时有乏力、头晕、心悸等不适，形寒肢冷，喜暖喜按。刻下症见双膝关节疼痛，伴下蹲、蹲起困难，平地行走时出现间歇性跛行，跛行距离不定。纳寐可，二便调。

History of present illness: The patient had bilateral knee pain ten years ago, which was worse when she went upstairs and downstairs. Squatting was restricted. OA was diagnosed at other hospital but not properly treated, leading to recurrent pain which was aggravated by exertion but relieved by rest. Ten months ago, due to sharp knee pain, she had difficulty walking during which intermittent claudication occurred with varying claudication distance. Discomforts like fatigue, dizziness and palpitation sometimes appear. She had cold limbs. The pain could be relieved by heat and pressure.

Current symptoms: Pain in the knees, restricted squatting, intermittent claudication during walking on the flat ground with variable claudication distance, good appetite, restful sleep, normal urination frequency and regular bowel movements.

目诊：勒答上白睛浅淡，龙脉脉络弯曲。甲诊：甲色苍白，半月痕暴露少。壮医诊断：骆芡－阴证－正虚型。中医诊断：骨痹病－肝肾亏虚证。

Eye examination: The white of the eyes is pale. The blood vessels of the eyes are curved.

Nail examination: The nails are pale with small fingernail lunulae.

Diagnosis in ZM:"Luoqian" characterized by insufficiency of the healthy qi, a type of yin deficiency.

Diagnosis in TCM: Bone impediment characterized by liver-kidney deficiency syndrome.

治疗：壮医药物竹罐疗法结合壮药内服治疗。

Treatment method: Apply the ZM bamboo cupping therapy and take Zhuang herbal medicinals.

处方如下。

Prescription.

（1）壮医药物竹罐疗法。部位：双膝部位各 10 罐（隔日 1 次）。

(1) The ZM bamboo cupping therapy. Applied areas: Respectively put 10 cups on and around each knee, one time every other day.

（2）壮药内服。处方：狗脊 15 g，扶芳藤 15 g，鸡血藤 15 g，当归藤 15 g，宽筋藤 15 g。6 剂，每日 1 剂，每剂水煎至 450 mL，分早中晚 3 次饭后温服。

(2) Zhuang herbal medicinals for oral administration. Prescription: Gouji (Rhizoma Cibotii) 15 g, Fufangteng (Caulis Euonymi Fortunei cum Foliis) 15 g, Jixueteng (Caulis Spatholobi) 15 g, Dangguiteng (*Embelia parviflora* Wall.) 15 g and Kuanjinteng (Caulis Tinosporae Sinensis) 15 g. Decoct one dose of the medicinals with water to 450 mL daily and take the warm decoction 3 times a day after meals, 6 doses is a treatment course.

二诊（2021 年 1 月 7 日）：经壮医药物竹罐疗法治疗 3 次、服药 6 剂后，患者双膝关节疼痛缓解，能下蹲，可拄拐自行行走，纳寐可，二便调，睡眠、饮食均佳，继服上方 3 剂，巩固疗效。

Second visit (on January 7, 2021): The knee pain was relieved after the ZM bamboo cupping therapy had been applied 3 times, combined with six-day of Zhuang herbal decoction taking. The patient had been able to squat and walk with a stick. She reported good appetite, restful sleep, normal urination frequency and regular bowel movements. The patient was instructed to take the same decoction for another 3 days to consolidate the efficacy.

按语：骆芡缘于患者年老体虚，感受风毒、湿毒、寒毒，阻滞三道两路，使天、地、人三气不能同步而致病。本案患者症见双膝关节疼痛，伴下蹲、蹲起困难，平地行走时可出现间歇性跛行，跛行距离不定，纳寐可，二便调。舌质淡，苔薄白，脉沉细。目诊见勒答上白睛浅淡，龙脉脉络弯曲。甲诊见甲色苍白，半月痕暴露少，五诊合参，本病病机为龙路、火路运行不畅，故关节疼痛，屈伸不利。舌质淡、苔薄白、脉沉细为正虚之征，故证属阴证－正虚型，兼有瘀毒，病位在关节。

Summary statement: As a type of OA ("Luoqian" in ZM), the patient's disease occurred due to weak constitution caused by aging. Under such circumstances, her body was attacked by wind, cold and dampness, which blocked the three passages and two channels. The blockage made the heaven-qi, earth-qi and human-qi unable to be synchronized, leading to the onset of the disease. On the first visit, the patient reported knee pain with restricted squatting, intermittent claudication during walking on the flat ground with variable claudication distance, good appetite, restful sleep, normal urination frequency and regular bowel movements. Her tongue was pale with white, thin coating. Her pulse was deep and thready. The white of her eyes was pale, and the blood vessels on her eyes were curved. Her fingernails were pale with small fingernail lunulae. By means of the five diagnostic methods[*], the mechanism of the disease was the blockage of the dragon and fire channels, which led to knee pain and loss of joint flexibility. Her pale tongue with white, thin coating and deep, thready pulse signified insufficiency of the healthy qi, a type of yin deficiency, accompanied by blood stasis. The disease sites were in her joints.

本案治疗以壮医外治与壮药内服相结合。外治法采用壮医药物竹罐疗法施于双膝部，以达疏通龙路火路、补肝肾、消肿痛之效。内服方中狗脊性温，味苦、

---

* The five diagnostic method refers to examination of tongue, eye and nail, inspection and pulse palpation.

甘，祛风毒，除湿毒，强腰膝，通龙路，为主药，有补肝肾、壮筋骨、祛风湿的功效。扶芳藤味微苦，性微温，益气血，补肝肾，舒筋活血；当归藤味苦、涩，性温，活血散瘀，补肾强腰，为帮药。宽筋藤、鸡血藤味微苦，性微寒，通火路，祛风毒，除湿毒，止疼痛，为带药。诸药配伍，共奏祛风毒、散寒毒之功。

Accordingly, the disease was treated with the ZM bamboo cupping therapy, which was applied to the knees, and oral administration of Zhuang herbal medicinals. The ZM bamboo cupping therapy is used to relax tendons, unblock the dragon and fire channels, tonify the liver and kidney and relieve swelling and pain. In terms of the herbal medicinals, Gouji (Rhizoma Cibotii) is bitter and sweet in taste and warm in nature. It can dispel wind and remove dampness, strengthen the lower back and knees, and unblock the dragon channel. It is used as the sovereign drug in formula with other drugs to tonify the liver and kidney, strengthen muscles and bones, dispel wind and remove dampness. Fufangteng (Caulis Euonymi Fortunei cum Foliis) and Dangguiteng (*Embelia parviflora* Wall.) are used as the minister drug. Fufangteng (Caulis Euonymi Fortunei cum Foliis) is a little bitter in taste and slightly warm in nature. It can replenish qi and blood, tonify the liver and kidney, relax tendons and activate blood. Dangguiteng (*Embelia parviflora* Wall.) is bitter and astringent in taste and warm in nature. It can activate blood, dispel stasis, tonify the kidney and strengthen the lower back. As the envoy drug, Kuanjinteng (Caulis Tinosporae Sinensis) and Jixueteng (Caulis Spatholobi) are a little bitter in taste and slightly cold in nature. They can unblock the fire channel, dispel wind and remove dampness, and relieve pain. They are used with other drugs to dispel wind and dissipate cold.

【病案二】

［Case 2］

陈某，女，84岁，2021年1月22日初诊。

Patient: Chen, an 84-year-old woman; her first visit was on January 22, 2021.

主诉：双膝疼痛10年余，加重2天。

Chief complaint:"I have had bilateral knee pain for more than ten years, which was worse two days ago."

现病史：患者10余年前出现双膝疼痛，久行久站加重，休息缓解，上下楼梯、下蹲困难。曾于医院住院，查双膝 X 射线提示双膝关节退行性病变。诊断为双侧膝关节骨性关节病，经治疗病情好转后出院。2 天前天气变冷后双膝关节疼痛加重，以右膝、右腘窝为甚，伴腰部胀痛、左下肢麻痛，屈伸、行走困难，不能下蹲。

History of present illness: The patient had bilateral knee pain more than 10 years ago, which was aggravated by a prolonged walking and standing but relieved by rest. The patient was once admitted to our hospital because she was diagnosed with "bilateral knee osteoarthropathy" due to degeneration of knee joints shown by the X-ray examination of both knees. She was discharged from the hospital after treatment. Two days ago, the pain in knees increased as the temperature decreased, especially in the right knee and popliteal fossa. The pain was accompanied by a distending pain in the lower back and a numb pain in the left lower limb. She reported decreased knee flexion and extension, walking difficulty and inability to squat.

目诊：勒答上白睛浅淡，龙脉脉络弯曲、末端有瘀点。甲诊：甲色苍白，半月痕暴露少。壮医诊断：骆芡－阴证－正虚型。中医诊断：双侧膝关节骨性关节病。

Eye examination: The white of the eyes is pale. The blood vessels of the eyes are curved with petechiae on the ends.

Nail examination: The nails are pale with small fingernail lunulae.

Diagnosis in ZM:"Luoqian" characterized by insufficiency of the healthy qi, a type of yin syndrome.

Diagnosis in TCM: Bilateral knee osteoarthropathy.

治疗：壮医药物竹罐疗法结合壮药内服治疗。

Treatment method: Apply the ZM bamboo cupping therapy and take Zhuang herbal medicinals.

处方如下。

Prescription.

（1）壮医药物竹罐疗法。部位：双膝部位 20 罐（隔日 1 次）。

(1) The ZM bamboo cupping therapy. Applied areas: Put 20 cups on and around the knees, one time every other day.

（2）壮药内服。处方：狗脊 15 g，桑寄生 20 g，鸡血藤 15 g，当归藤 15 g，杜仲藤 15 g，宽筋藤 15 g。7 剂，每日 1 剂，每剂水煎至 450 mL，分早中晚 3 次饭后温服。

(2) Zhuang herbal medicinals for oral administration. Prescription: Gouji (Rhizoma Cibotii) 15 g, Sangjisheng (Ramulus Taxilli) 20 g, Jixueteng (Caulis Spatholobi) 15 g, Dangguiteng (*Embelia parviflora* Wall.) 15 g, Duzhongteng (Cortex Parabarii) 15 g and Kuanjinteng (Caulis Tinosporae Sinensis) 15 g. Decoct one dose of the medicinals with water to 450 mL daily and take the warm decoction 3 times a day after meals, 7 doses is a treatment course.

二诊（2021 年 1 月 29 日）：经壮医药物竹罐疗法治疗 3 次、服药 7 剂后，患者双膝疼痛缓解，可自行屈伸、行走，仍不能下蹲，二便调，纳可，寐欠佳，继续采用壮医药物竹罐疗法，内服方中加夜交藤、酸枣仁安神。

Second visit (on January 29, 2021): The pain in the knees was relieved after the ZM bamboo cupping therapy had been applied three times, combined with seven-day of Zhuang herbal decoction taking. The patient was able to bend and straighten her knees, and walk but still unable to squat. She reported good appetite, normal urination frequency and regular bowel movements but restless sleep. Therefore, the ZM bamboo cupping therapy continues to be applied. In terms of oral administration, for tranquilizing the mind, Yejiaoteng (Caulis Polygoni Multiflori) and Suanzaoren (Semen Ziziphi Spinosae) were added.

三诊（2021 年 2 月 5 日）：经治疗后，患者双膝疼痛缓解，下蹲改善，可拄拐自行，纳寐可，二便调。

Third visit (on February 5, 2021): After treatment, the knee pain was further relieved. The patient could squat and walk with a stick. She reported good appetite, restful sleep, normal urination frequency and regular bowel movements.

按语: 骆芡缘于患者年老体虚，受伤留瘀，感受邪毒（风毒、寒毒、湿毒等），客于筋骨，阻滞龙路、火路，使天、地、人三气不能同步而致病。本案患者症见双膝疼痛，右膝为甚，右侧腘窝牵扯痛，屈伸、行走困难，不能下蹲，腰部胀痛，左下肢麻痛。舌质暗红，苔少，脉沉细。目诊见勒答上白睛浅淡，龙脉脉络弯曲、末端有瘀点。五诊合参，本病缘于患者年老体虚，风毒、湿毒乘虚而入，阻滞三道两路，使天、地、人三气不能同步而发病。气血运行不畅，故关节疼痛。舌质暗红、苔少、脉沉细为正虚之征，故证属阴证－正虚型，兼有瘀毒，病位在关节。

Summary statement: OA ("Luoqian" in ZM) often occurs in people with weak constitution due to aging or with blood stasis after injury. Under such circumstances, the body tends to be attacked by pathogenic toxins such as wind, cold and dampness. Subsequently, the static blood and pathogenic toxins stagnate in tendons and bones and then block the dragon and fire channels. The blockage makes the heaven-qi, earth-qi and human-qi unable to be synchronized, leading to the onset of the disease. On the first visit, the patient reported pain in the knees, especially in the right knee and popliteal fossa, decreased knee flexion and extension, walking difficulty, inability to squat, a distending pain in the lower back and a numb pain in the left lower limb. Her tongue was dark red with little coating. Her pulse was deep and thready. The white of her eyes was pale and the blood vessels of her eyes were curved with petechiae at the ends. By means of the five diagnostic methods, it is confirmed that as a type of "Luoqian" (OA), the patient's disease occurred because pathogenic toxins such as wind and dampness attacked her body due to weak constitution which was caused by aging. The toxins blocked the three passages and two channels. Subsequently, the blockage made the heaven-qi, earth-qi and human-qi unable to be synchronized, leading to the onset of the disease. Unsmooth movement of qi and blood led to pain in joints. Her dark red tongue with a little coating and deep, thready pulse signified insufficiency of the healthy qi with blood stasis, a type of yin deficiency. The disease site was in her joints.

本案治疗以壮医外治与壮药内服相结合。外治法采用壮医药物竹罐疗法施于双侧膝部以疏通龙路、火路，消肿痛。内服方中狗脊、桑寄生性温，味苦、甘，祛风毒，除湿毒，强腰膝，通龙路，合为主药。鸡血藤味苦、微甘，性微热，调龙路、火路，补血虚，除湿毒；当归藤、杜仲藤活血散瘀，补肾强腰，共为帮药，奏祛风毒散寒毒之功。宽筋藤微苦，性微寒，通火路，祛风毒，除湿毒，止疼痛，为带药。诸药配伍，共奏补肾壮骨、祛风毒、除湿毒之功。

Accordingly, the disease was treated with the ZM bamboo cupping therapy, which was applied to the knees, and oral administration of Zhuang herbal medicinals. The ZM bamboo cupping therapy is used to unblock the dragon and fire channels, and relieve swelling and pain. In terms of the herbal medicinals, Gouji (Rhizoma Cibotii) and Sangjisheng (Ramulus Taxilli) are bitter and sweet in taste and warm in nature. As the sovereign drug, they can dispel wind and remove dampness, strengthen the lower back and knees and unblock the dragon channel. Jixueteng (Caulis Spatholobi) is bitter and little sweet in taste and hot in nature. It can regulate the dragon and fire channels, tonify blood deficiency and remove dampness. As the minister drug, Dangguiteng (*Embelia parviflora* Wall.) and Duzhongteng (Cortex Parabarii) can activate blood, remove blood stasis and tonify the kidney to strengthen the lower back. They can be used with other herbs to dispel wind and dissipate cold. As the envoy drug, Kuanjinteng (Caulis Tinosporae Sinensis) is a little bitter in taste and slightly cold in nature. It can unblock the fire channel, dispel wind and remove dampness, and relieve pain. It can also be used with other drugs to dispel wind and dissipate cold.

【病案三】

［Case 3］

郑某，女，61 岁，2021 年 2 月 27 日初诊。

Patient: Zheng, a 61-year-old woman; her first visit was on February 27, 2021.

主诉：双膝反复疼痛 5 年，加重 1 年。

Chief complaint:"I have had recurrent bilateral knee pain for more than five years, which was worse one year ago."

现病史：患者自诉于 5 年前出现双膝关节反复疼痛，伴下蹲、蹲起受限，未系统诊疗，症状反复，劳累后加重，休息可缓解。自发病以来，形寒肢冷，喜暖，遇寒痛增，得热痛减，时有双膝屈伸不利，行走困难，偶感乏力，无关节晨僵、变形，无口干、眼干、牙齿片状脱落、腮腺肿大，无反复发热、口腔溃疡、光过敏、雷诺现象等，神清，精神尚可，纳寐可，二便调。体重未见明显变化。刻下症见左膝疼痛，活动后加重。

History of present illness: The patient reported she had bilateral knee pain more than five years ago, which was accompanied by restricted squatting. She did not have proper treatment so the symptoms were recurrent. The pain was aggravated by exertion but relieved by rest. Since the disease occurred, she had cold limbs. The intolerance of cold could be relieved by heat. The falling temperature increases the pain while the rising temperature decreases it. Sometimes, she had difficulty in bending and straightening her knees, and walking. Occasionally, she felt weak. No morning joint stiffness, joint deformity, dry mouth or eye dryness. Her teeth were not lost. Her bilateral parotid glands were not enlarged. No recurrent fever, oral ulcers, photosensitivity or Raynaud's phenomenon. She reported a clear state of mind, good spirits, good appetite, restful sleep, normal urination frequency and regular bowel movements, and stable weight.

Current symptoms: Pain in her left knee, which gets worse by exertion.

目诊：勒答上白睛浅淡，龙脉脉络弯曲。甲诊：甲色苍白，半月痕暴露过少。壮医诊断：骆芡－阴证－正虚型。西医诊断：双侧膝关节骨性关节病。

Eye examination: The white of the eyes is pale. The blood vessels of the eyes are curved.

Nail examination: The nails are pale with small fingernail lunulae.

Diagnosis in ZM:"Luoqian" characterized by insufficiency of the healthy qi, a type of yin syndrome.

Diagnosis in WM: Bilateral knee osteoarthropathy.

治疗：壮医药物竹罐疗法结合壮药内服治疗。

Treatment method: Apply the ZM bamboo cupping therapy and take Zhuang herbal medicinals.

处方如下。

Prescription.

（1）壮医药物竹罐疗法。部位：双膝部位 10 罐（隔日 1 次）。

(1) The ZM bamboo cupping therapy. Applied areas: Put 10 cups on and around the knees, one time every other day.

（2）壮药内服。处方：狗脊 15 g，桑寄生 20 g，当归藤 15 g，杜仲藤 10 g，宽筋藤 15 g。3 剂，每日 1 剂，每剂水煎至 450 mL，分早中晚 3 次饭后温服。

(2) Zhuang herbal medicinals for oral administration. Prescription: Gouji

(Rhizoma Cibotii) 15 g, Sangjisheng (Ramulus Taxilli) 20 g, Dangguiteng (*Embelia parviflora* Wall.) 15 g, Duzhongteng (Cortex Parabarii) 15 g and Kuanjinteng (Caulis Tinosporae Sinensis) 15 g. Decoct one dose of the medicinals with water to 450 mL daily and take the warm decoction 3 times a day after meals, 3 doses is a treatment course.

二诊（2021 年 3 月 2 日）：经壮医药物竹罐疗法治疗 3 次、服药 3 剂后，患者双膝时有隐痛，二便正常，睡眠、饮食均佳，继行上法，加强疗效。

Second visit (on March 2, 2021): After the ZM bamboo cupping therapy had been applied three times, combined with three-day of decoction taking, dull pain in knees occurred sometimes. The patient reported good appetite, restful sleep, normal urination frequency and regular bowel movements. She was instructed to take the same decoction for another four days to consolidate the efficacy.

三诊（2021 年 3 月 7 日）：经治疗后，患者双膝关节疼痛好转，能下蹲，二便正常，睡眠、饮食均佳。

Third visit (on March 7, 2021): After treatment, the bilateral knee pain was significantly relieved. The patient was able to squat. She reported good appetite, restful sleep, normal urination frequency and regular bowel movements.

按语：骆芡缘于患者年老体虚，受伤留瘀，感受邪毒（风毒、寒毒、湿毒等），客于筋骨，阻滞龙路、火路，使天、地、人三气不能同步而致病。本案患者症见左膝疼痛，活动后加重。目诊见勒答上白睛浅淡，龙脉脉络弯曲。甲诊见甲色苍白，半月痕暴露过少。五诊合参，本病属于骆芡范畴，缘于患者年老体虚，感受风毒、湿毒、寒毒，或外伤留瘀，阻滞三道两路，使天、地、人三气不能同步而致病。正气亏虚，气血不足，骨、筋肉、关节失养，故见关节酸累，沉重，疼痛，肢体乏力；或伴形寒肢冷、喜按喜暖，甚则关节变形，屈伸不利，行走困难，乏力。舌质淡、苔薄白、脉沉细为正虚之征。病性属虚，病位在肝肾、关节。

Summary statement: OA ("Luoqian" in ZM) often occurs in people with weak constitution due to aging or with blood stasis after injury. Under such circumstances, the body tends to be attacked by pathogenic toxins such as wind, cold and dampness. Subsequently, the static blood and toxins stagnate in tendons and bones and then block the dragon and fire channels. The blockage makes the heaven-qi, earth-qi and human-qi unable to be synchronized, leading to the onset of the disease. On the first visit, the patient reported pain in her left knee, which was worse by exertion. Her tongue was pale with white, thin coating. The white of her eyes was pale and the blood vessels of her eyes were curved. Her nails were pale with small fingernail lunulae. By means of the five diagnostic methods, it is confirmed that the patient's disease, as a type of "Luoqian" (OA) occurred due to her weak constitution or blood stasis after injury. Under such circumstances, pathogenic toxins such as wind, cold and dampness attacked her body. These toxins with static blood blocked the three passages and two channels, leading to the failure of synchronization of the heaven-qi, earth-qi and human-qi. As a result, the healthy qi and blood were insufficient, and bones, muscles and joints weren't provided with adequate nourishment. This resulted in soreness, heaviness and pain in her joints, limb weakness, cold limbs, joint deformity, decreased joint flexibility, and walking difficulty. The tolerance of cold was relieved by heat and pressure. Her pale tongue with white, thin coating and her deep, thready pulse signified insufficiency of the healthy qi, a type of deficiency syndrome. The disease sites were in her liver, kidney and joints.

　　本案治疗以壮医外治与壮药内服相结合。外治法采用壮医药物竹罐疗法施于左膝部以疏通龙路火路，消肿痛。内服方中狗脊味苦、甜，性温，补阳虚，强腰膝，祛风毒，除湿毒；桑寄生味苦、甘，性平，祛风湿，利关节，通龙路、火路，壮筋骨，合为主药。当归藤味苦、涩，性温，活血散瘀，补肾强腰；杜仲藤味苦、微辛，性平，祛风活络，散瘀止痛，强筋壮骨，合为帮药，增强其壮筋骨、补气血之力。宽筋藤味微苦，性微寒，通火路，祛风毒，除湿毒，止疼痛，辛温走窜，为带药。诸药合用，以壮筋骨、补气血为主，兼祛风毒、散寒毒，使正虚得补，风毒得解，寒毒被清，湿毒得除，龙路、火路得以疏通。

Accordingly, the disease was treated with the ZM bamboo cupping therapy, which was applied to the left knee, and oral administration of Zhuang herbal medicinals. The ZM bamboo cupping therapy is used to unblock the dragon and fire channels, and relieve swelling and pain. In terms of the herbal medicinals, Gouji (Rhizoma Cibotii) is bitter and sweet in taste and warm in nature. It can replenish yang deficiency, strengthen the lower back and knees, and dispel wind and remove dampness. Sangjisheng (Ramulus Taxilli) is bitter and sweet in taste and neutral in nature. It can expel wind, remove dampness and benefit joints. These two herbs can be used together as the sovereign drug to unblock the dragon and fire channels, and strengthen muscles and bones. Dangguiteng (*Embelia parviflora* Wall.) is bitter and astringent in taste and warm in nature. It can activate blood, dispel stasis, tonify the kidney to strengthen the lower back. Duzhongteng (Cortex Parabarii) is bitter and slightly spicy in taste and neutral in nature. It can dispel wind, activate couaterals, remove blood stasis, relieve pain, and strengthen muscles and bones. These two herbs can be used as the minister drug to strengthen muscles and bones, and tonify qi and blood. As the envoy drug, Kuanjinteng (Caulis Tinosporae Sinensis) is a little bitter in taste and slightly cold in nature. It can unblock the fire channel, dispel wind and remove dampness, and relieve pain. All the herbal medicinals take the synergistic effect to strengthen muscles and bones, tonify the healthy qi and blood, remove wind, cold and dampness and unblock the dragon and fire channels.

（二）滚克（类风湿关节炎）

2　Rheumatoid Arthritis ("Gunke" in ZM)

1. 疾病概述

2.1　General description

滚克属于壮医发旺（风湿病）范畴，多缘于患者身体虚弱，邪毒（风毒、湿毒、寒毒、痧毒等）乘虚而入，阻滞龙路、火路，使天、地、人三气不能同步，风寒湿毒客于肢体关节，气血运行不畅而致病。以小关节疼痛、肿胀、晨僵为特点。相当于中医的尪痹、西医的类风湿关节炎。

From the perspective of ZM, as a type of "Fawang" (rheumatic diseases in WM), "Gunke", also known as lameness impediment in TCM and rheumatoid arthritis in WM, often occurs in people with weak constitution. Under such circumstances, the body tends to be attacked by pathogenic toxins such as wind, dampness, cold and filth, which block the dragon and fire channels. The blockage makes the heaven-qi, earth-qi and human-qi unable to be synchronized. Concurrently, the stagnation of the toxins at the joints leads to unsmooth movement of qi and blood. As a result, the disease occurs. It is characterized by tenderness, swelling and morning stiffness in small joints.

类风湿关节炎是临床上常见的一种慢性、进行性、侵蚀性的自身免疫系统疾病，具有较高的发病率和致残率。患者一般先出现滑膜组织炎症，疾病进行性发展，逐渐出现关节软骨及骨质破坏，最终可能发展为关节畸形，导致功能障碍，给患者的健康及生活质量带来严重不利影响（图6、图7）。

Rheumatoid arthritis (RA) is a common chronic, progressive and erosive autoimmune disease with high morbidity and disability. Initially, the synovium becomes inflamed. As RA progresses, synovial inflammation causes cartilage and bone destruction, which ultimately leads to joint deformity and functional decline (Fig. 6 and Fig. 7). Consequently, patients' health and quality of life will be seriously affected.

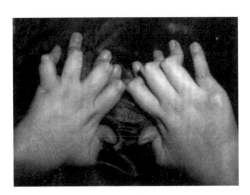 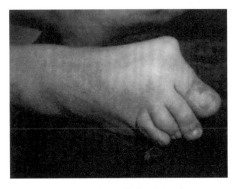

图6 类风湿关节炎手部改变　　　　　图7 类风湿关节炎足部改变
Fig.6 Hand deformity due to RA　　　　Fig.7 Foot deformity due to RA

2. 病因病机

2.2 Cause and mechanism of disease

滚克属于壮医发旺（风湿病）范畴，多缘于患者身体虚弱，邪毒（风毒、湿毒、寒毒、痧毒等）乘虚而入，阻滞龙路、火路，使天、地、人三气不能同步，风寒湿毒客于肢体关节，气血运行不畅而致病。以小关节疼痛、肿胀、晨僵为特点。

From the perspective of ZM, as a type of "Fawang" (rheumatic diseases in WM),

"Gunke", also known as lameness impediment in TCM and rheumatoid arthritis in WM, often occurs in people with weak constitution. Under such circumstances, the body tends to be attacked by pathogenic toxins such as wind, dampness, cold and filth, which block the dragon and fire channels. The blockage makes the heaven-qi, earth-qi and human-qi unable to be synchronized. Concurrently, the stagnation of the toxins at the joints leads to unsmooth movement of qi and blood. As a result, the disease occurs. It is characterized by tenderness, swelling and morning stiffness in small joints.

3. 诊查要点

2.3　Essentials for diagnosis

（1）主症。小关节呈对称性疼痛肿胀，多发于手指关节，出现晨僵、屈伸不利等症状，严重者伴肌肉筋骨酸痛、麻木乏力，后期关节变形，活动困难。

(1) Main symptoms. Symmetrical pain and swelling, morning stiffness, flexion and extension negative in small joints, more commonly in finger joints. For the severe disorder, an aching pain, numbness and weakness occur in muscles, tendons and bones, ultimately leading to joint deformity and difficulty moving.

（2）兼症。怕风，发热，口渴，烦闷，身重，全身乏力，睡眠差，腹胀，少数病例有皮下结节。

(2) Concurrent symptoms. Aversion to wind, fever, thirst, vexation, heavy sensation of the body, general debility, restless sleep and abdominal distension, sometimes subcutaneous nodules in a few patients.

（3）目诊。勒答上白睛浅淡，或白睛有雾斑或瘀斑，龙脉脉络散乱，或脉络弯曲、暗红或红活。

(3) Eye examination. The white of the eyes is pale, on which there may be cloudy or blood spots. The blood vessels on the eyes have stretched or are curved in dark or bright red.

（4）甲诊。症轻者甲色淡红，症重者甲色深红、青紫或苍白，半月痕暴露过多或过少。

(4) Nail examination. The nails of patients with mild RA are light red while those of patients with severe RA are dark red, bluish purple or pale, with small or

large fingernail lunulae.

（5）本病起病缓慢，反复迁延不愈，患者逐渐形体消瘦，且常因感受风寒湿邪而病情反复。

(5) RA has a slow onset, which is persistent and recurrent. It causes the constitution that gradually become emaciated. Invasion of wind, cold and/or dampness is a major cause for its recurrence.

（6）血液中类风湿因子（RF）阳性或增高，活动期 C-反应蛋白（CRP）、血沉（ESR）增高。

(6) A higher level of rheumatoid factor (RF) is detected in blood. The values of C-reactive protein (CRP) and erythrocyte sedimentation rate (ESR) are higher.

（7）X 射线摄影胶片可见骨质疏松改变，或关节骨面侵蚀等。

(7) X-ray image shows osteoporosis or articular bone erosion.

4. 辨证论治

2.4　Syndrome differentiation and treatment

（1）治疗原则。祛风除湿，活血舒筋，散寒止痛，拔毒消肿，通龙路、火路气机。

(1) Treatment principles. Dispel wind, remove dampness, activate blood, relax tendons, dissipate cold, relieve pain, draw out toxins to eliminate swelling, and move qi in the dragon and fire channels.

（2）适宜证型。适用于阳证、阴证伴有瘀毒者。

(2) Indications. Yang syndrome or yin syndrome with blood stasis.

（3）壮药。选用肿节风、伸筋草等。

(3) Zhuang herbal medicinals. Zhongjiefeng (Herba Sarcandrae), Shenjincao (Herba Lycopodii), etc.

（4）治疗部位或穴位。以局部阿是穴为主，再视关节病变情况取邻近穴位。局部阿是穴主要选取关节疼痛或肿胀的部位。邻近穴位包括肩关常穴（肩髃、肩贞、肩前）、肘关常穴（曲池、肘髎、曲泽）、腕关常穴（阳池、大陵、外关）、掌指关常穴（合谷、中渚、腕骨）、髋关常穴（环跳、髀关、居髎）、膝关常穴（鹤顶、足三里、阴陵泉、阳陵泉）、踝关常穴（解溪、冲阳、丘墟）、跖趾关常穴（太冲、内庭、足临泣）。

(4) Acupoints selection. Select Ashi points on the affected area as the primary ones and take adjacent points as secondary ones if necessary. Specifically, select Ashi points on the painful or swollen joint areas and adjacent points, including Jianyu (LI 15), Jianzhen (SI 9), Jianqian (EX-UE 12), Quchi (LI 11), Zhouliao (LI 12), Quze (PC 3), Yangchi (TE 4), Daling (PC 7), Waiguan (TE 5), Hegu (LI 4), Zhongzhu (TE 3), Wangu (SI 4), Huantiao (GB 30), Biguan (ST 31), Juliao (GB 29), Heding (EX-LE 2), Zusanli (ST 36), Yinlingquan (SP 9), Yanglingquan (GB 34), Jiexi (ST 41), Chongyang (ST 42), Qiuxu (GB 40), Taichong (LR 3), Neiting (ST 44) and Zulinqi (GB 41).

（5）具体操作步骤如前述。

(5) The process of treatment for RA is the same as that described in Paragraph 2.5 (The cupping process) of Section Ⅲ.

5. 预防调护

2.5　Prevention and care

（1）饮食调理。饮食宜清淡，多食富含胶质和钙的食物。忌食肥甘厚味及辛辣之品。中晚期偏虚者可适当滋补。阳证宜食清热毒、化湿毒之品，如薏苡仁、红豆等，食疗方可用薏苡排骨冬瓜汤、鸡矢藤莲子鸭汤等。阴证宜食祛风毒、散寒毒、除湿毒、调气补虚的血肉有情之品，如山药、陈皮，食疗方可用山药羊肉炖黑豆汤等。

(1) Dietary adjustments. A diet low in fat and salt but high in colloid and calcium is preferable. Greasy, sweet, salty and spicy foods are forbidden. In moderate or end-stage RA, patients with deficiency syndrome should eat nutritious foods as appropriate. Patients with yang syndrome are recommended to eat foods that clear away heat and remove dampness, such as the coix seed and red bean. Recommended dietary supplements are pork ribs soup with wax gourd and coix seed, duck soup with Jishiteng (Herba Paederiae) and lotus seeds, etc. Patients with yin syndrome are recommended to eat foods that dispel wind, dissipate cold and remove dampness, adjust qi and reinforce deficiency, such as yam and dried tangerine peel. A recommended dietary supplement is lamb soup with yam and black bean.

（2）生活起居。注意保暖，避风寒、劳逸结合，避免劳累。

(2) Daily life. Patients should keep themselves warm, and balance rest and work.

（3）情志调摄。帮助患者正确认识病情、了解治疗方法、过程及锻炼方法，树立战胜疾病的信心。

(3) Emotional adjustments. Patients should understand RA, the treatment procedure and exercises for it, which will help them to establish confidence in curing it.

（4）关节功能锻炼。活动期应注意休息，减少活动量，尽量将病变关节固定于功能位，如膝关节、肘关节应尽量伸直。缓解期应及时注意关节功能锻炼，如慢步、游泳可锻炼全身关节功能，握握力器或捏核桃可锻炼手指关节功能，双手握转环旋转可锻炼腕关节功能，脚踏自行车可锻炼膝关节功能，滚圆木、踏空缝纫机可锻炼踝关节功能等。

(4) Joint mobility exercises. Patients should use the affected joints less and keep them in their functional positions, for example, keep knee and elbow joints straight as the patients can. Patients with RA in remission should do exercises to improve joint function, for example, logging and swimming for all body joints, using a hand gripper or pinching walnut for hand joints, rotating a rotating ring with two hands for wrist joints, cycling for knee joints, and logrolling and moving feet in a one-up-one-down pedal motion for ankle joints.

6. 医案选读

2.6　Selected case readings

【病案一】

［Case 1］

王某，男，58 岁，2021 年 1 月 22 日初诊。

Patient: Wang, a 58-year-old man; his first visit was on January 22, 2021.

主诉：四肢多关节反复肿痛 20 年，加重 20 天。

Chief complaint:"I have had recurrent swelling and pain in my multiple extremity joints for 20 years, which became worse 20 days ago."

现病史：患者 20 年前以双手掌指关节、近端指间关节肿痛起病，伴双手晨僵，持续时间超过 1 小时。当地医院查 RF 阳性，诊断为类风湿关节炎，治疗后缓解（具体用药不详）。平时未规律服药治疗，关节肿痛症状反复，逐渐累及双肘、双肩、双踝、双膝关节，关节肿痛明显时自服止痛药治疗，症状可减轻。7 年前患者曾至壮医医院就诊，查 RF 30 IU/mL，ESR 33 mm/h，诊断同前。予壮医外治、壮药内服，用雷公藤多苷片、正清风痛宁缓释片抗风湿治疗，病情好转。平时未服药治疗，关节肿痛时有反复，可耐受。20 天前患者出现右踝、左膝肿痛，症状逐渐加重，影响行走活动。症见右踝、左膝关节肿痛、灼热，舌质红，苔黄腻，脉弦滑。

History of present illness: Twenty years ago, pain and swelling occurred in the metacarpophalangeal and proximal interphalangeal joints of the hands, which were accompanied by morning stiffness of the hands that lasted more than one hour. RA was diagnosed by the positive RF test done at a local hospital. It was in remission after treatment (specific medication unknown). Patient did not take his regular medication so pain and swelling reappeared and gradually travelled up to bilateral elbow and shoulder joints and down to bilateral knee and ankle joints. These symptoms could be alleviated by taking painkillers. Seven years ago, the patient sought medical care at our hospital. The diagnosis was the same as before by a RF test (30 IU/mL) and ESR test (33 mm/h). Therefore, he was given the ZM external treatment combined with oral administration of tripterygium wilfordii polyglycosides tablets and Zhengqing Fengtongning sustained-release tablets. Afterwards, his symptoms were relieved. However, he did not take his medications onwards so the pain and swelling were recurrent but tolerable. Twenty days ago, worsening pain and swelling in his right ankle and left knee joints caused walking difficulty.

Current symptoms: Pain, swelling and a burning sensation in the joints of the right ankle and left knee, red tongue with yellow, greasy coating, and wiry, slippery pulse.

目诊：勒答上龙脉脉络弯曲、红活。甲诊：甲色深，半月痕暴露多。壮医诊断：滚克－阳证－湿热型。中医诊断：尪痹－湿热阻痹。

Eye examination: The blood vessels on the eyes are curved and reddened.

Nail examination: The nails are black with large fingernail lunulae.

Diagnosis in ZM:"Gunke" characterized by dampness-heat syndrome, a type of yang syndrome.

Diagnosis in TCM: Dampness-heat impediment, a type of lameness impediment.

治疗：壮医药物竹罐疗法结合壮药内服治疗。

Treatment method: Apply the ZM bamboo cupping therapy and take Zhuang herbal medicinals.

处方如下。

Prescription.

（1）壮医药物竹罐疗法。部位：双膝、双踝部位 20 罐（隔日 1 次）。

(1) The ZM bamboo cupping therapy. Applied areas: Respectively put 20 cups on and around the knees and ankles, one time every other day.

（2）壮药内服。处方：肿节风 20 g，救必应 10 g，两面针 9 g，伸筋草 15 g。3 剂，每日 1 剂，每剂水煎至 450 mL，分早中晚 3 次饭后温服。

(2) Zhuang herbal medicinals for oral administration. Prescription: Zhongjiefeng (Herba Sarcandrae) 20 g, Jiubiying (Cortex Ilicis Rotundae) 10 g, Liangmianzhen (Radix Zanthoxyli) 9 g and Shenjincao (Herba Lycopodii) 15 g. Decoct one dose of the medicinals with water to 450 mL daily and take the warm decoction 3 times a day after meals, 3 doses is a treatment course.

二诊（2021 年 1 月 30 日）：经壮医药物竹罐疗法治疗 3 次、服药 3 剂后，患者左膝、右踝关节疼痛缓解，无肿胀，能自行行走，二便正常，睡眠、饮食均佳。

Second visit (on January 30, 2021): After the ZM bamboo cupping therapy had been applied 3 times, combined with three-day of decoction taking, pain in the patient's left knee and right ankle joints was relieved, without swelling. He could walk on his own. He reported good appetite, restful sleep, normal urination frequency and regular bowel movements.

按语：滚克属于壮医发旺（风湿病）范畴，多缘于患者身体虚弱，邪毒（风毒、湿毒、寒毒、痧毒等）乘虚而入，阻滞龙路、火路，使天、地、人三气不能同步，风寒湿邪客于肢体关节，气血运行不畅而致病。以小关节疼痛、肿胀、晨僵为特点。本案患者症见右踝、左膝关节肿痛、灼热，舌质红，苔黄腻，脉弦滑，勒答上龙脉脉络弯曲、红活，甲色深，半月痕暴露多。五诊合参，本病属于壮医学滚克范畴，缘于患者身体虚弱，邪毒（风毒、湿毒、热毒等）乘虚而入，阻滞龙路、火路，使天地人三气不能同步，风湿毒客于肢体关节，气血运行不畅而致病。舌质红、苔黄腻、脉弦滑为湿热之征，证属于阳证（湿热型）。

Summary statement: From the perspective of ZM, as a type of "Fawang" (rheumatic diseases in WM), "Gunke" (rheumatoid arthritis in WM) often occurs in people with weak constitution. Under such circumstances, the body tends to be attacked by pathogenic toxins such as wind, dampness, cold and filth, which block the dragon and fire channels. The blockage makes the heaven-qi, earth-qi and human-qi unable to be synchronized. Concurrently, the stagnation of the toxins at the joints leads to unsmooth movement of qi and blood. As a result, the disease occurs. It is characterized by tenderness, swelling and morning stiffness in small joints. On the first visit, the patient reported pain, swelling and a burning sensation in the joints of his right ankle and left knee. His tongue was red with yellow, greasy coating. His pulse was wiry and slippery. The blood vessels of his eyes were curved and reddened. His nails were black with large fingernail lunulae. By means of the five diagnostic methods, it is confirmed that the patient's disease is a type of "Gunke". It occurred due to his weak constitution. Under such circumstances, his body was attacked by pathogenic toxins such as wind, dampness and cold, which blocked the dragon and fire channels. The blockage made the heaven-qi, earth-qi and human-qi unable to be synchronized. Concurrently, the stagnation of the toxins at the joints led to unsmooth movement of qi and blood, resulting in the onset of the disease. His red tongue with yellow, greasy coating and wiry, slippery pulse signified dampness-heat syndrome, a type of yang syndrome.

本案治疗以壮医外治与壮药内服相结合，外治法采用壮医药物竹罐疗法以清热毒，除湿毒，通调龙路火路，消肿止痛。壮药内服以清热毒、除湿毒、祛风毒为治法，方中肿节风味苦、微辛，性平，为解湿毒要药，具有除湿毒、祛风毒、化瘀血、消肿痛的功效，为主药。救必应性寒，味苦，清热毒，除湿毒，消肿止痛；两面针味辛、苦，性平，祛风活血，止痛消肿，二药合用，共为帮药，协同主药增强祛风毒、除湿毒、通络止痛的功效。伸筋草是性微温之品，通调龙路、火路，增强除湿毒、止疼痛的功效，为带药。本方以主帮带合用，使热毒得清，湿毒得除，风毒得解，龙路、火路得以疏通，筋络关节肿痛得以消除。

Accordingly, the disease was treated with the ZM bamboo cupping therapy and oral administration of Zhuang herbal medicinals. The ZM bamboo cupping therapy is used to clear away heat, remove dampness and dispel wind, regulate the dragon and fire channels, eliminate swelling and relieve pain. In terms of the herbal medicinals, they serve the same treatment purpose as the external therapy. Zhongjiefeng (Herba Sarcandrae) is bitter and slightly spicy in taste and neutral in nature. It is used as the sovereign drug to remove dampness and dispel wind, and resolve blood stasis, relieve pain and eliminate swelling. Jiubiying (Cortex Ilicis Rotundae) is bitter in taste and cold in nature. It can clear away heat and remove dampness, eliminate swelling and relieve pain. Liangmianzhen (Radix Zanthoxyli) is spicy and bitter in taste and slightly warm in nature. It can dispel wind, activate blood, relieve pain and eliminate swelling. As the minister drug, these two herbs are used with the sovereign drug to enhance the efficacy of dispelling wind and removing dampness and unblocking collaterals to relieve pain. As the envoy drug, Shenjincao (Herba Lycopodii) is slightly warm in nature. It can regulate the dragon and fire channels, enhance the ability of other herbs in the formula to remove dampness, and relieve pain. In this formula, the sovereign, minister and envoy drugs are combined to clear away heat, remove dampness and dispel wind, and unblock the dragon and fire channels to treat swelling and pain in joints.

【病案二】

［Case 2］

林某，女，68岁，2021年2月19日初诊。

Patient: Lin, a 68-year-old woman; her first visit was on February 19, 2021.

主诉：四肢关节反复对称性肿痛11年，加重1个月。

Chief complaint:"I have had recurrent symmetrical pain and swelling in my multiple extremity joints for 11 years, which became worse one month ago."

现病史：患者11年前出现双手近端指间、双手掌指、双肘、双肩、双肩关节等四肢多关节肿痛，呈持续性、对称性，伴双手晨僵，持续时间长于1小时，伴有关节活动受限，反复发作。查RF、抗环瓜氨酸肽（CCP）抗体高滴度阳性，CRP、ESR升高，关节彩色多普勒超声检查提示滑膜炎，确诊为类风湿关节炎。先后服用雷公藤多苷片、甲氨蝶呤等药物治疗，症状减轻，但反复发作，劳累、阴雨天为甚。刻下症见双腕、双肘肿痛，双肩疼痛。舌质红，苔黄腻，脉滑数。

History of present illness: Symmetrical pain and swelling in multiple extremity joints, including metacarpophalangeal and proximal interphalangeal joints of the hands and joints of elbows and shoulders, have been going on for 11 years. In addition, morning stiffness of the hands lasts more than one hour and joint flexibility has decreased. These symptoms were recurrent. The colour Doppler ultrasonography revealed synovitis, but combined with the positive RF test, anti-CCP positivity at high titer, raised CRP and ESR levels, the disease was diagnosed as RA. After the patient had taken tripterygium wilfordii polyglycosides tablets and methotrexate, the symptoms were relieved, but reappeared and became worse after exertion or on rainy days.

Current symptoms: Pain in the wrists, elbows and shoulders, accompanied by swelling in her wrists and elbows. Her tongue is red with yellow, greasy coating. Her pulse is slippery and rapid.

目诊：勒答上龙脉脉络弯曲。甲诊：甲色深红，半月牙暴露过多。壮医诊断：滚克－阳证－湿热型。中医诊断：尪痹－湿热阻痹。

Eye examination: The blood vessels on the eyes are curved.

Nail examination: The nails are dark red with large fingernail lunulae.

Diagnosis in ZM:"Gunke" characterized by dampness-heat syndrome, a type of yang syndrome.

Diagnosis in TCM: Dampness-heat impediment, a type of lameness impediment.

治疗：壮医药物竹罐疗法治疗。

Treatment method: Apply the ZM bamboo cupping therapy.

部位：双肩、双肘部 20 罐（隔日 1 次）。

Applied areas: Put 20 cups respectively on and around the shoulders and elbows, one time every other day.

二诊（2021 年 2 月 23 日）：经壮医药物竹罐疗法治疗 3 次、内服清热除湿壮药 6 剂，双肩、双肘关节疼痛减轻，无肿胀，上抬、外展仍受限，纳寐可，二便调。继行前法，加强巩固疗效。

Second visit (on February 23, 2021): After the ZM bamboo cupping therapy had been applied three times, combined with six doses of Zhuang herbal medicinals taking that clear away heat and remove dampness, the pain was relieved in the joints of the patient's shoulders and elbows, without swelling. But he still had difficulty in raising his arms up and out to the sides. He reported good appetite, restful sleep, normal urination frequency and regular bowel movements. He was treated with the previous therapeutic methods to consolidate the efficacy.

三诊（2021年3月1日）：经壮医药物竹罐疗法治疗3次、内服清热除湿壮药7剂后，双肩、双肘关节疼痛减轻，无肿胀，无活动受限，纳寐可，二便调。

Third visit (on March 1, 2021): After the ZM bamboo cupping therapy had been applied another three times, combined with seven doses of Zhuang herbal medicinals that clear away heat and remove dampness, the pain in the joints of the shoulders and elbows was further relieved. No swelling or joint movement limitations. He reported good appetite, restful sleep, normal urination frequency and regular bowel movements.

按语：滚克属于壮医发旺（风湿病）范畴，多缘于患者身体虚弱，邪毒（风毒、湿毒、寒毒、痧毒等）乘虚而入，阻滞龙路、火路，使天、地、人三气不能同步，风寒湿邪客于肢体关节，气血运行不畅而致病。以小关节疼痛、肿胀、晨僵为特点。本案患者症见双腕、双肘肿痛，双肩疼痛。舌质红，苔黄腻，脉滑数。目诊见勒答上龙脉脉络弯曲。甲诊见甲色深红，半月痕暴露过多。五诊合参，本病属于壮医滚克范畴，缘于毒邪客于关节，郁久化热，故见关节疼痛、肿胀，触之灼热或有热感。舌质红、苔黄腻、脉滑数为湿热之征，故证属阳证（湿热型）。治疗予壮医药物竹罐疗法祛风毒、清热毒、除湿毒、消肿痛，通畅三道两路。

Summary statement: From the perspective of ZM, as a type of "Fawang" (rheumatic diseases in WM), "Gunke" often occurs in people with weak constitution. Under such circumstances, the body tends to be attacked by pathogenic toxins such as wind, dampness, cold and filth, which block the dragon and fire channels. The blockage makes the heaven-qi, earth-qi and human-qi unable to be synchronized. Concurrently, the stagnation of the toxins at the joints leads to unsmooth movement of qi and blood. As a result, the disease occurs. It is characterized by tenderness, swelling and morning stiffness in small joints.

On the first visit, the patient reported pain in his wrists, elbows and shoulders, accompanied by swelling in his wrists and elbows. His tongue was red with yellow, greasy coating. His pulse was slippery and rapid. The blood vessels of his eyes were curved. His nails were black with large fingernail lunulae. By means of the five diagnostic methods, it is confirmed that the patient's disease is a type of "Gunke". It occurred because toxic pathogens stagnated in the joints and thus transformed to heat, leading to pain and swelling in joints where there was a burning or heat sensation. Her red tongue with yellow, greasy coating and slippery, rapid pulse signified dampness-heat syndrome, a type of yang syndrome. Therefore, the bamboo cupping therapy was used to clear away heat, remove dampness and dispel wind, eliminate swelling, relieve pain, unblock the three passages and two channels.

【病案三】

［Case 3］

周某，女，74 岁，2021 年 3 月 5 日初诊。

Patient: Zhou, a 74-year-old woman; her first visit was on March 5, 2021.

主诉：四肢多关节反复肿痛 3 月余。

Chief complaint:"I have had recurrent swelling and pain in my multiple extremity joints for more than 3 months."

现病史：患者 2020 年 11 月中旬出现双手近端指间关节、掌指关节肿痛，双手晨僵，持续约 3 分钟，活动后可缓解，遇寒痛增，得热痛减。未行相关检查，咨询风湿专科医生后考虑为类风湿关节炎，口服双蚁祛湿通络胶囊、雷公藤多苷片祛风湿止痛，美洛昔康抗炎止痛，关节肿痛无明显缓解，逐渐累及双腕、双膝、双踝，伴随双膝、双踝酸软乏力。症见双手近端指间关节、掌指关节肿痛，伴晨僵，双膝、双踝酸软乏力，右手背肿胀、灼热，右上臂疼痛，活动受限。舌质淡红，苔白腻，脉滑。

History of present illness: Pain and swelling occurred in the metacarpophalangeal and proximal interphalangeal joints of her two hands in mid-November 2020. Hand morning stiffness lasted about three minutes and could be relieved by exercises. The pain was increased by cold but reduced by heat. Without any examinations, the patient's medical conditions were considered as RA by merely consulting a rheumatologist. Subsequently, she took Shuangyi Qushi Tongluo capsules and tripterygium wilfordii polyglycosides tablets to dispel wind, remove dampness, relieve pain and meloxicam to treat pain and inflammation. However, these medications did not work properly. The pain and swelling travelled up to her wrist joints and down to her bilateral knee and ankle joints, accompanied by soreness and weakness in her knees and ankles.

Current symptoms: Pain, swelling and morning stiffness in the metacarpophalangeal and proximal interphalangeal joints of the hands, soreness and weakness in the knees and ankles, swelling and a burning sensation in the back of the right hand, pain in the right upper arm with movement limitation, reddish tongue with white and greasy coating, slippery pulse.

目诊：勒答上白睛浅淡，龙脉脉络弯曲、延伸。甲诊：甲色淡，半月痕暴露少。壮医诊断：滚克－阴证－寒湿型。中医诊断：尪痹－风寒湿痹。

Eye examination: The white of the eyes is pale. The blood vessels of the eyes are curved and stretched.

Nail examination: The nails are pale with small fingernail lunulae.

Diagnosis in ZM:"Gunke" characterized by cold-dampness syndrome, a type of yin syndrome.

Diagnosis in TCM: Wind-cold-dampness impediment, a type of lameness impediment.

治疗：壮医药物竹罐疗法结合壮药内服治疗。

Treatment method: Apply the ZM bamboo cupping therapy and take Zhuang herbal medicinals.

处方如下。

Prescription.

（1）壮医药物竹罐疗法。部位：双膝、双肩部各 10 罐（隔日 1 次）。

(1) The ZM bamboo cupping therapy. Applied areas: Respectively put 10 cups on and around each knee and shoulder, one time every other day.

（2）壮药内服。处方：半枫荷 20 g，大风艾 10 g，九龙藤 20 g，海风藤 15 g，丢了棒 15 g。6 剂，每日 1 剂，每剂煎成 450 mL，分早中晚饭后温服。

(2) Zhuang herbal medicinals for oral administration. Banfenghe (Radix

Pterospermi Heterophylli) 20 g, Dafeng'ai (Folium et Cacumen Blumeae Balsamiferae) 10 g, Jiulongteng (Radix seu Caulis Bauhiniae Championii) 20 g, Haifengteng (Caulis Piperis Kadsurae) 15 g and Diulebang (Claoxylon Indicum) 15 g. Decoct one dose of the medicinals with water to 450 mL daily and take the warm decoction 3 times a day after meals, 6 doses is a treatment course.

二诊（2021 年 3 月 16 日）：经壮医药物竹罐疗法治疗 4 次、服药 6 剂后，患者双膝、右上臂疼痛缓解，右上肢活动受限，双踝酸软乏力，纳寐可，二便调。继续予以壮医药物竹罐疗法治疗，内服方加杜仲、牛膝补益肝肾。

Second visit (on March 16, 2021): After the ZM bamboo cupping therapy had been applied 4 times, combined with six-day of decoction taking, pain in the patient's knees and right upper arm was relieved but the movement of her right upper limb was still limited and her ankles were sore and weak. She reported good appetite, restful sleep, normal urination frequency and regular bowel movements. Therefore, the bamboo cupping therapy continued to be applied. In terms of oral administration, for tonifying the liver and kidney, Duzhong (Cortex Eucommiae) and Niuxi (Radix Achyranthis Bidentatae) were added.

三诊（2021 年 3 月 24 日）：经治疗后，患者双膝、双踝、双上肢无明显疼痛、肿胀。无乏力，纳寐可，二便调。

Third visit (on March 24, 2021): The patient reported apparent relief of pain and swelling in her knees, ankles and upper limbs, no soreness or weakness, good appetite, restful sleep, normal urination frequency and regular bowel movements.

按语：滚克属于壮医发旺（风湿病）范畴，多缘于患者身体虚弱，邪毒（风毒、湿毒、寒毒、痧毒等）乘虚而入，阻滞龙路、火路，使天、地、人三气不能同步，风寒湿邪客于肢体关节，气血运行不畅而致病。以小关节疼痛、肿胀、晨僵为特点。本案患者症见双手近端指间关节、掌指关节肿痛，伴晨僵，双膝、双踝酸软乏力，右手背肿胀、灼热，右上臂疼痛，活动受限。勒答上白睛浅淡，龙脉脉络弯曲、延伸。甲色淡，半月痕暴露少。舌质淡红，苔白腻，脉滑。五诊合参，本病属于壮医学滚克范畴，缘于患者年老体虚，不慎感受风毒、湿毒，阻滞龙路、火路，使天、地、人三气不能同步，素体虚弱，风寒湿毒客于肢体关节，气血运行不畅而致病。三道两路不通，故关节肿痛，屈伸不利。舌质红、苔白腻、脉滑为风寒湿之征。故证属阴证，病位在关节，病性为毒。

Summary statement: From the perspective of ZM, as a type of "Fawang" (rheumatic diseases in WM), "Gunke" often occurs in people with weak constitution. Under such circumstances, the body tends to be attacked by pathogenic toxins such as wind, dampness, cold and filth, which block the dragon and fire channels. The blockage makes the heaven-qi, earth-qi and human-qi unable to be synchronized. Concurrently, the stagnation of the pathogenic toxins at the joints leads to unsmooth movement of qi and blood. As a result, the disease occurs. It is characterized by tenderness, swelling and morning stiffness in small joints.

On the first visit, the patient reported pain, swelling and morning stiffness in the metacarpophalangeal and proximal interphalangeal joints of her hands, soreness and weakness in her knees and ankles, swelling and a burning sensation in the back of her right hand, pain in her right upper arm with movement limitation. The white of her eyes was pale and the blood vessels of her eyes were curved and stretched. Her nails were pale with small fingernail lunulae. Her tongue was reddish with white, greasy coating. Her pulse was slippery. By means of the five diagnostic methods, it is confirmed that the patient's disease, as a type of "Gunke", occurred due to her weak constitution. Under such circumstances, her body was attacked by pathogenic toxins such as wind and dampness, which blocked the dragon and fire channels. The blockage made the heaven-qi, earth-qi and human-qi unable to be synchronized. Concurrently, the stagnation of the pathogenic toxins at the joints led to unsmooth movement of qi and blood, resulting in the onset of the disease. Her reddish tongue with white, greasy coating and slippery pulse signified wind-cold-dampness syndrome, a type of yin syndrom. The sites of the disease, which was toxic in nature, were in her joints.

本案治疗以壮医外治与壮药内服相结合，外治法采用壮医药物竹罐疗法，散寒毒，除湿毒，止痹痛，通调龙路火路，消肿止痛。壮药内服以散寒毒、除湿毒、温经通络为法。方中半枫荷味甘淡，性微温，长于祛风寒之毒、除在里之湿毒并活血消肿；大风艾性微温，味辛、苦，助祛风寒毒之效，调经活血，二者共为主药。九龙藤味甘、性温，擅长祛风毒，除湿毒，通调龙路、火路，行气止痛；海风藤味苦、辣，性平，二者共为帮药，以助祛风湿之毒。丢了棒为味苦、性平之品，能祛风除湿，最擅舒经通脉止痛，故为带药。本方以主帮带合用，使寒毒得解，湿毒得除，龙路、火路得温则行，筋络关节痛止。

Accordingly, the disease was treated with the ZM bamboo cupping therapy and oral administration of Zhuang herbal medicinals. The ZM bamboo cupping therapy is used to dispel cold and remove dampness, eliminate arthralgia, regulate the dragon and fire channels to eliminate swelling and relieve pain. In terms of the herbal medicinals, they serve the same treatment purpose as the external therapy. Banfenghe (Radix Pterospermi Heterophylli) is slightly sweet in taste and slightly warm in nature. It is excellent at dispelling wind and cold. It can also remove dampness and activates blood to eliminate swelling. Dafeng'ai (Folium et Cacumen Blumeae Balsamiferae) is bitter and spicy in taste and slightly warm in nature. It can dispel wind and cold, regulate menstruation and activate blood. These two herbs are used as the sovereign drug. Jiulongteng (Radix seu Caulis Bauhiniae Championii) is sweet in taste and warm in nature. It can dispel wind and remove dampness, regulate the dragon and fire channels to move qi and relieve pain. Haifengteng (Caulis Piperis Kadsurae) is bitter and spicy in taste and neutral in nature. It can dispel wind and remove dampness. These two herbs are used as minister drug. Diulebang (Claoxylon Indicum) is bitter in taste and neutral in nature. In addition to dispelling wind and removing dampness, it is excellent at unblocking the meridians and promoting blood circulation to relieve pain, so it is often used as the envoy drug. In this formula, the sovereign, minister and envoy drugs are combined to dispel wind, dissipate cold and remove dampness and warm the dragon and fire channels to move qi in them, resulting in relief of pain in tendons and joints.

（三）令扎（强直性脊柱炎）

3　Ankylosing spondylitis ("Lingzha" in ZM)

1. 疾病概述

3.1　General description

令扎属于壮医发旺（风湿病）范畴，缘于患者先天禀赋不足，身体虚弱，邪毒（风毒、湿毒、寒毒、热毒、痧毒等）乘虚而入，阻滞三道两路，使天、地、人三气不能同步而致病。主要临床表现为腰背疼痛、四肢关节疼痛、肿胀、晨僵、屈伸不利等。相当于中医的大偻、西医的强直性脊柱炎。

From the perspective of ZM, as a type of "Fawang" (rheumatic diseases in WM), "Lingzha", also known as "Dalou" in TCM and ankylosing spondylitis in WM, often occurs in people with congenital defect or weak constitution. Under such circumstances, the body is vulnerable to invasion of pathogenic toxins such as wind, dampness, cold, heat and filth, which block the three passages and two channels. The blockage will make the heaven-qi, earth-qi and human-qi unable to be synchronized, leading to the onset of the disease. The clinical manifestations include tenderness in the lumbar region and the back, and tenderness, swelling, morning stiffness in the limb joints with flexion and extension negative.

强直性脊柱炎是一种慢性进行性炎性疾病，主要侵犯骶髂关节、脊柱骨突、脊柱旁软组织、外周关节及肌腱、韧带附着于骨的部位，常引起纤维性和骨性强直。本病以腰背疼痛、双髋活动受限、严重者脊柱弯曲变形甚至强直僵硬为临床特点。本病患者多为 10～40 岁，男性好发且患病症状重，进展快。在我国患病率为 0.26%，给患者家庭和社会带来沉重的负担。

Ankylosing spondylitis (AS) is a chronic progressive inflammatory disease. It causes inflammation in the sacroiliac joints, spinal condyles, paraspinal soft tissues, peripheral joints, and tendons and ligaments attached to bones, resulting in fibrous ankylosis and bone ankylosis. It is characterized by tenderness in the lumbar region and the back, and reduced range of motion of the hips, spinal deformity and ankylosis which occur in people with severe ankylosing spondylitis. Age at onset of AS typically peaks between the age of 10 and 40. Men are more likely than women to develop AS. In addition, its severity is higher and progression is faster. The prevalence of AS in China is approximately 0.26%, causing a massive impact on patients' families and society.

2. 病因病机

3.2　Cause and mechanism of disease

本病多缘于患者先天禀赋不足，身体虚弱，邪毒（风毒、湿毒、寒毒、热毒、痧毒等）乘虚而入，阻滞三道两路，使天、地、人三气不能同步而致病。

AS often occurs in people with congenital defect or weak constitution. Under such circumstances, the body is vulnerable to invasion of pathogenic toxins such as wind, dampness, cold, heat and filth, which block the three passages and two channels. The blockage will make the heaven-qi, earth-qi and human-qi unable to be synchronized, leading to the onset of the disease.

3. 诊查要点

3.3　Essentials for diagnosis

（1）主症。以腰骶部疼痛为主，或有髋、肩等四肢关节疼痛，重者可出现背脊弯曲、屈伸不利、活动障碍等。

(1) Main symptoms: Pain primarily occurs in the lumbosacral region, which may be accompanied by pain in limb joints. Severe AS can cause the abnormal curvature in the spine, flexion and extension negative and movement disorders.

（2）兼症。伴膝腿乏力，腰脊僵困，或喜暖畏寒，见寒加重，得热则舒，或性情急躁，低热，喜见凉爽等。

(2) Concurrent symptoms: Weakness in the knees and legs and stiffness in the lumbar region and spine; preference for heat and aversion to cold with the symptoms which are aggravated by cold and relieved by heat; or impatience, low-grade fever and preference for cool, etc.

（3）目诊。勒答上龙脉脉络曲张，或见血管末端有瘀点。多见于青少年。

(3) Eye examination: The blood vessels of the eyes are twisted and enlarged, or with petechiae on the ends. The symptoms are more often seen in adolescence with the disease.

（4）X射线检查。提示单侧骶髂关节炎或双侧骶髂关节炎。

(4) X-ray examination: Unilateral or bilateral sacroiliac arthritis.

4. 辨证论治

3.4　Syndrome differentiation and treatment

（1）治疗原则。祛风除湿，活血舒筋，散寒止痛，拔毒消肿，通龙路、火路气机。

(1) Treatment principles. Dispel wind, remove dampness, activate blood, relax

tendons, dissipate cold, relieve pain, draw out toxins to eliminate swelling, and move qi in the dragon and fire channels.

（2）适宜证型。适用于阳证、阴证伴有瘀毒者。

(2) Indications: Yang syndrome and yin syndrome with blood stasis.

（3）壮药。选用杜仲藤、海风藤等。

(3) Zhuang herbal medicinals: Duzhongteng (Cortex Parabarii), Haifengteng (Caulis Piperis Kadsurae), etc.

（4）治疗部位或穴位。以局部阿是穴为主，再视关节病变情况取邻近穴位。关常穴包括腰背关常穴（夹脊、肾俞、腰阳关、腰俞、上髎、次髎、中髎）、颈关常穴（大椎、颈百劳）、髋关常穴（环跳、髀关、居髎）、肘关常穴（曲池、肘髎、曲泽）、膝关常穴（鹤顶、阴陵泉、阳陵泉、足三里、犊鼻、委中）、踝关常穴（解溪、冲阳、丘墟、昆仑）、跖趾关常穴（太冲）。

(4) Selection of acupoints: Select Ashi points on the affected area as the primary ones and take adjacent points as secondary ones if necessary. Commonly used acupoints include cervical and lumbar Jiaji (EX-B 2), Shenshu (BL 23), Yaoyangguan (GV 3), Yaoshu (GV 2), Shangliao (BL 31), Ciliao (BL 32), Zhongliao (BL 33), Dazhui (GV 14), Jingbailao (EX-HN 15), Huantiao (GB 30), Biguan (ST 31), Juliao (GB 29), Quchi (LI 11), Zhouliao (LI 12), Quze (PC 3), Heding (EX-LE 2), Yinlingquan (SP 9), Yanglingquan (GB 34), Zusanli (ST 36), Dubi (ST 35), Weizhong (BL 40), Jiexi (ST 41), Chongyang (ST 42), Qiuxu (GB 40), Kunlun (BL 60) and Taichong (LR 3).

5. 预防调护

3.5　Prevention and care

（1）纠正患者的不良站姿、坐姿，告诫患者行走、站、坐都要保持良好的姿态，保证腰背的正常生理曲度，降低脊柱畸形发生的可能性。

(1) Correct patients' standing and sitting postures and ask them to maintain a good posture while walking, standing and sitting to keep the natural curves of the spine and lower the risk of developing a spinal deformity.

（2）注意睡眠姿势。提醒患者在睡眠时可多变换几次体位，以促进全身血液循环，缓解晨僵；早晨醒后，可在床上轻微活动或揉搓按摩容易发生僵硬的肢体关节部位，以改善局部血流，放松肌肉，起床后再行肢体屈伸、腰背扭转等活动，能使晨僵尽快缓解。日常生活中，注意不要长时间保持同一体位坐、站、卧，体位改变时，动作要轻缓，以免摔跤而致骨折。

(2) Suggestions: Change sleep position to boost the whole-body blood circulation and relieve morning stiffness. After waking up in the morning, do light exercises or massage the limb joints prone to be stiff on the bed to improve local blood flow and relax muscles. After getting up, perform activities, for example, bending and stretching the limbs, twisting the lower back, to relieve morning stiffness as soon as possible. Do not sit, stand, or lie in the same position for a long time, and change the position slowly to prevent falls and fractures.

（3）坚持进行肢体锻炼，尤其是腰背、髋部运动，保持腰背及各关节的生理活动度。建议做康复操，每日 2 次。同时建议游泳锻炼，并持之以恒。

(3) Ask patients to do regular exercises for the limbs, especially for the lumbar region, back and hips, to maintain the normal range of motion of the lumbar region, back and joints. Recommend patients to do rehabilitation exercises twice daily and insist on swimming.

6. 医案选读

3.6　Selected case readings

【病案一】

［Case 1］

梁某，男，34 岁，2021 年 8 月 12 日初诊。

Patient: Liang, a 34-year-old man; his first visit was on August 12, 2021.

主诉：腰背僵痛 3 年，加重 4 天。

Chief complaint:"I have had stiffness and pain in my lumbar region and back for 3 years, which became worse 4 days ago."

现病史：患者诉 2018 年无明显诱因下出现腰背部僵痛、弯腰困难，晨起为甚，久坐后加重，活动后缓解，当时患者未予重视及诊疗。2019 年 8 月患者腰背僵痛加重，至桂林医学院附属医院就诊，查腰椎磁共振成像（MRI）提示两侧骶髂关节异常改变，符合强直性脊柱炎改变，诊断为强直性脊柱炎，予注射用重组人 II 型肿瘤坏死因子受体－抗体融合蛋白 25 mg qw（每周 1 次）治疗，治疗后患者腰痛症状稍减轻。2019 年 12 月发现患肝癌后停药至今，停药后症状加重，活动受限明显，疼痛难忍时自服止痛药后症状减轻，但仍反复。症见腰背部、颈部、双肩部僵痛，活动受限，纳寐可，二便调。舌质红，苔黄，脉滑。

History of present illness: The patient reported stiffness and pain in the lumbar region and back with bending difficulty, which was worse when he woke up in the morning, occurred in 2018 without any apparent reasons. The symptoms were aggravated by prolonged sitting but relieved by exercises. He did not give much attention to the medical conditions and did not seek medical care. In August 2019, he sought medical care at the Affiliated Hospital of Guilin Medical University because the symptoms deteriorated. AS was diagnosed based on the MRI examination which showed abnormal changes in bilateral sacroiliac joints. Accordingly, he was treated with a once-a-week injection of 25 mg of recombinant human tumor necrosis factor receptor type II-antibody fusion protein. Afterwards, the pain in the lumbar region was slightly relieved. However, the treatment terminated in December 2019 when he was diagnosed with liver cancer. Consequently, the stiffness and pain in the lumbar region and back became worse, with greatly reduced range of motion. When the pain was unbearable, he took painkillers to relieve it temporarily.

Current symptoms: Pain and stiffness in the lumbar region, back, neck and shoulders, with reduced range of motion, good appetite, restful sleep, normal urination frequency and regular bowel movements, red tongue with yellow coating and slippery pulse.

目诊：勒答上龙脉脉络弯曲、红活，末端有瘀点。甲诊：甲色深红，半月痕暴露过多。中医诊断：脊痹病（大偻）－肾虚湿热证。壮医诊断：令扎－阳证。西医诊断：强直性脊柱炎。

Eye examination: The blood vessels of the eyes are curved and reddened with petechiae on the ends.

Nail examination: The nails are dark red with large fingernail lunulae.

Diagnosis in ZM:"Lingzha" characterized by yang syndrome.

Diagnosis in TCM: Spine impediment characterized by kidney deficiency with dampness-heat.

Diagnosis in WM: AS。

治疗：壮医药物竹罐疗法结合壮药内服治疗。

Treatment method: Apply the ZM bamboo cupping therapy and take Zhuang herbal medicinals.

处方如下。

Prescription.

（1）壮医药物竹罐疗法。部位：双膝、双肩部各 10 罐（隔日 1 次）；颈部、腰部关常穴 20 罐。隔日 1 次，10 ～ 14 天为 1 个疗程。

(1) The ZM bamboo cupping therapy. Applied areas: Respectively put 20 cups on and around each knee and shoulder, one time every other day; put 20 cups on each of commonly used acupoints on the neck and lower back, one time every other day, 10~14 days is a treatment course.

（2）壮药内服。处方：忍冬藤 15 g，桑枝 15 g，骨碎补 15 g，槲寄生 15 g，杜仲藤 9 g，两面针 9 g。6 剂，每日 1 剂，每剂水煎至 300 mL，分早中晚 3 次分服。

(2) Zhuang herbal medicinals for oral administration. Prescription: Rendongteng (Caulis Lonicerae Japonicae) 15 g, Sangzhi (Ramulus Mori) 15 g, Gusuibu (Rhizoma Drynariae) 15 g, Hujisheng (Herba Visci) 15 g, Duzhongteng (Cortex Parabarii) 9 g and Liangmianzhen (Radix Zanthoxyli) 9 g. Decoct one dose of the medicinals with water to 300 mL daily and take the warm decoction 3 times a day after meals, 6 doses is a treatment course.

二诊（2021 年 8 月 18 日）：经壮医药物竹罐疗法治疗 3 次配合服药 6 剂后，患者腰背部、颈部、双肩部僵痛稍减轻，继行壮医药物竹罐疗法（腰部 20 罐）。内服药在原方上加炒僵蚕 10 g 祛风通络止痛，黄花倒水莲 20 g 补气虚、除湿毒、疏通龙路火路止痛。

Second visit (on August 18, 2021): After the ZM bamboo cupping therapy had been applied three times, combined with six-day of decoction taking, pain and stiffness in the lumbar region, back, neck and shoulders was slightly relieved. Therefore, the bamboo cupping therapy continued to be applied to the lower back with 20 cups. In terms of oral administration, for dissipating wind, unblocking collaterals and relieving pain, 10 g of stir-baked Jiangcan (Bombyx Batryticatus) were added; for tonifying qi, removing dampness, unblocking the dragon and fire channels to relieve pain, 20 g of Huanghuadaoshuilian (Radix seu Folium Polygalae Fallacis) were added.

三诊（2021 年 8 月 24 日）患者腰背部、颈部、双肩部僵痛较前减轻。壮医外治疗法同前。内服药在原方上加白芍、白术、砂仁缓急止痛，健脾和胃。14 剂，每日 3 次，每次 150 mL，饭后温服。

Third visit (on August 24, 2021): Stiffness and pain in the patient's lumbar region, back, neck and shoulders was further relieved. Therefore, the same external therapy was applied. In terms of oral administration, for relaxing spasm and relieving pain, invigorating the spleen and harmonizing the stomach, Baishao (Radix Paeoniae Alba), Baizhu (Rhizoma Atractylodis Macrocephalae) and Sharen (Fructus Amomi) were added. One dose of the medicinals was decocted in water daily and 150 mL of the warm decoction was taken 3 times a day after meals, 14 doses is a treatment course.

按语：强直性脊柱炎常见于青年男性，属壮医令扎范畴，缘于患者先天禀赋不足，身体虚弱，风毒、湿毒、热毒乘虚而入，阻滞三道两路，使天、地、人三气不能同步而发病。气血运行不畅，故关节疼痛。舌质红、苔黄、脉滑为阳证之征。故证属阳证，病位在关节。

Summary statement: From the perspective of ZM, the patient's disease, AS which is often seen in young men, is a type of "Lingzha". Such type often occurs in people with congenital defect or weak constitution. Under such circumstances, the body is vulnerable to invasion of wind, dampness and heat, which block the three passages and two channels. The blockage will make the heaven-qi, earth-qi and human-qi unable to be synchronized, resulting in the onset of the disease. Unsmooth movement of qi and blood leads to joint pain. Patients with such type of "Lingzha" usually have a red tongue with yellow coating and slippery pulse, which are the signs of yang syndrome and indicate that the disease sites are in joints.

治疗当达疏通龙路火路、祛风湿、除湿毒、止痹痛的功效，在治疗方法上多采用壮医药物竹罐疗法配合壮药内服的方法治疗。

Accordingly, the treatment should aim to unblock the dragon and fire channels, dispel wind, remove dampness and eliminate arthralgia. Therefore, the ZM bamboo cupping therapy combined with oral administration of Zhuang herbal medicinals is preferable.

本案患者患强直性脊柱炎病程较长，腰背部、颈部、双肩部僵痛，活动受限。舌质红，苔黄，脉滑，属阳证。治以疏通龙路火路、祛风湿、除湿毒、止痹痛，采用壮医药物竹罐疗法施于颈肩部、腰部以疏通龙路火路，疼痛可减。内服壮药重在清热毒，除湿毒，兼壮筋骨。方中忍冬藤、桑枝均为性寒之品，擅于清热毒，通调龙路，后者并能除湿毒，合为主药。槲寄生、骨碎补、杜仲藤均能祛风毒、除湿毒、壮筋骨、消肿痛，三者合为帮药。两面针性微温，味辛、苦，可通调龙路火路，为带药，引上药共奏祛风毒、除湿毒，强筋骨，消肿痛之功，使三气同步，气血得畅，筋骨得健。

The patient's disease lasted for a long time. Stiffness and pain occurred in his lumbar region, back, neck and shoulders, with reduced range of motion. His red tongue with yellow coating and slippery pulse signified yang syndrome. Therefore, the treatment for him aimed to unblock the dragon and fire channels, dispel wind, remove dampness and eliminate arthralgia. Accordingly, the ZM bamboo cupping therapy was applied to his neck, shoulders and lower back to relieve pain. The oral administration of Zhuang herbal medicinals aimed to clear away heat and remove dampness with due consideration to strengthening tendons and bones. Rendongteng (Caulis Lonicerae Japonicae) and Sangzhi (Ramulus Mori) are cold in nature, and can clear away heat and regulate the dragon channel. Besides, Sangzhi (Ramulus Mori) can remove dampness, so they are used as the sovereign drug. Gusuibu (Rhizoma Drynariae), Hujisheng (Herba Visci) and Duzhongteng (Cortex Parabarii) can remove dampness and dispel wind, strengthen tendons and bones, relieve pain and eliminate swelling, so they are used as the minister drug. As the envoy drug, Liangmianzhen (Radix Zanthoxyli) is spicy and bitter in taste and slightly warm in nature. It can regulate the dragon and fire channels. It can also be used with other drugs to remove dampness and dispel wind, strengthen tendons and bones, relieve pain and eliminate swelling, resulting in synchronization of the heaven-qi, earth-qi and human-qi, smooth movement of qi and blood, and strong tendons and bones.

【病案二】

［Case 2］

林某，男，38 岁，2021 年 2 月 20 日初诊。

Patient: Lin, a 38-year-old man; his first visit was on February 20, 2021.

主诉：腰部反复隐痛 14 年，加重 2 月余。

Chief complaint:"I have had a dull pain in my lower back for 14 years, which became worse 2 months ago."

现病史：患者 2007 年以腰部隐痛起病，未诊治，症状反复，但未加重。2017年患者感腰骶部疼痛较前明显，夜间及晨起为甚，伴晨僵，活动后逐渐减轻。外院查人类白细胞抗原 B27（HLA-B27）阳性，诊断为强直性脊柱炎。间断服用止痛药治疗，症状可缓解，但反复，并出现颈肩部疼痛，遂来诊治，予壮医外治并壮药内服，用重组人Ⅱ型肿瘤坏死因子受体－抗体融合蛋白 25 mg biw（每周 2 次）皮下注射控制病情，症状缓解，平时规律用药。2 月余前患者自行停药，逐渐出现左侧颈肩部、腰部、左髋部疼痛，纳寐一般，二便调，舌质红，苔薄黄，脉细。

History of present illness: The patient's disease started with a dull pain in his lower back in 2007. He did not have any treatment so the pain was recurrent but not worse. In 2017, he had obvious lumbosacral pain, especially at night and in the morning when he woke up. He also had morning stiffness that was relieved with exercises. He was diagnosed with AS at other hospital based on a positive HLA-B27 antigen test. The symptoms were relieved by taking painkillers intermittently but recurred. When neck and back pain occurred, he sought medical care at our department. He was treated with the ZM external therapy and oral administration of Zhuang herbal medicinals, combined with a twice-a-week injection of 25 mg of recombinant human tumor necrosis factor receptor type Ⅱ-antibody fusion protein. Afterwards, the symptoms were relieved. The patient had been having regular treatments until more than two months ago. Consequently, pain developed in the left side of his neck, left shoulder, lower back and left hip. He reported good appetite, restful sleep, normal urination frequency and regular bowel movements.

His tongue is red with yellow, thin coating. His pulse is thready.

目诊：勒答上龙脉脉络弯曲、延伸。甲诊：甲色深红，半月痕暴露过多。壮医诊断：令扎－阴证－肾虚型。中医诊断：脊痹病－肾虚湿热证。西医诊断：强直性脊柱炎。

Eye examination: The blood vessels of the eyes are curved and stretched.

Nail examination: The nails are dark red with large fingernail lunulae.

Diagnosis in ZM:"Lingzha" characterized by kidney deficiency syndrome, a type of yin syndrome.

Diagnosis in TCM: Kidney deficiency with dampness-heat syndrome, a type of spine impediment.

Diagnosis in WM: AS.

治疗：壮医药物竹罐疗法结合壮药内服治疗。

Treatment method: Apply the ZM bamboo cupping therapy and take Zhuang herbal medicinals.

处方如下。

Prescription.

（1）壮医药物竹罐疗法。部位：双侧颈肩部、腰部、右髋部等交替进行，隔1～2天1次，14天为1个疗程。

(1) The ZM bamboo cupping therapy. Applied areas: Put cups on both sides of the neck, the lower back or right hip, one time every 1~2 days, 14 days is a course of treatment.

（2）壮药内服。处方：忍冬藤20 g，伸筋草15 g，桑枝10 g，两面针10 g，杜仲藤10 g，槲寄生20 g，甘草6 g。7剂，每日1剂，每剂水煎至450 mL，分早中晚3次服用。

(2) Zhuang herbal medicinals for oral administration. Prescription: Rendongteng (Caulis Lonicerae Japonicae) 20 g, Shenjincao (Herba Lycopodii) 15 g, Sangzhi (Ramulus Mori) 10 g, Liangmianzhen (Radix Zanthoxyli) 10 g, Duzhongteng (Cortex Parabarii) 10 g, Hujisheng (Herba Visci) 20 g and Gancao (Radix et Rhizoma Glycyrrhizae) 6 g. Decoct one dose of the medicinals with water to 450 mL daily and take the warm decoction 3 times a day after meals, 7 doses is a treatment course.

二诊（2021年2月25日）：患者颈肩部、腰背部、双髋关节疼痛较前减轻，纳寐可，二便调。继服上方，巩固疗效。

Second visit (on February 25, 2021): Pain in the joints of the patient's neck, shoulders, lower back, back and hips was relieved. He reported good appetite, restful sleep, normal urination frequency and regular bowel movements. Therefore, he was instructed to continue taking the same decoction to consolidate the efficacy.

按语：强直性脊柱炎常见于青年男性，属于壮医令扎范畴，缘于患者先天禀赋不足，风毒、湿毒、热毒乘虚而入，阻滞三道两路，使天、地、人三气不能同步而发病。气血运行不畅，故关节疼痛，舌质红、苔薄黄、脉细为阳证之征。治疗上以补肾虚祛湿热为治病之本，多采用壮医药物竹罐疗法配合壮药内服的方法治疗。

Summary statement: From the perspective of ZM, the patient's disease, AS which is often seen in young men, is a type of "Lingzha". Such type often occurs in those with congenital defect which makes the body vulnerable to invasion of wind, dampness and heat, which blocks the three passages and two channels. The blockage will make the heaven-qi, earth-qi and human-qi unable to be synchronized, resulting in the onset of the disease. Unsmooth movement of qi and blood leads to joint pain. Patients with such type of "Lingzha" usually have a red tongue with yellow, thin coating and thready pulse, which are the signs of yang syndrome. Accordingly, the treatment should aim to tonify kidney deficiency, remove dampness and clear away heat, so the ZM bamboo cupping therapy combined with oral administration of Zhuang herbal medicinals is preferable.

本案患者患强直性脊柱炎病程较长，主要表现为反复腰部疼痛，休息时加重，活动后逐渐减轻。治宜以清热毒、除湿毒为主，兼壮筋骨。采用壮医药物竹罐疗法治疗颈肩部、腰部、右髋部以清热毒、除湿毒、通龙路火路、止痛。配合壮药内服，方中忍冬藤为性寒之品，擅于清热毒，通调龙路，为主药。槲寄生、杜仲藤均能祛风毒、除湿毒、壮筋骨、消肿痛；伸筋草味微苦、辣，性温，祛风毒，除湿毒，通龙路；三者合为帮药。两面针性微温，味辛、苦，可通调龙路火路；甘草调和诸药；二者共为带药。引上药共奏祛风毒、除湿毒、强筋骨、消肿痛之功，使三气同步，气血得畅，筋骨得健。

The patient's disease lasted for a long time. It was characterized by recurrent pain in his lumbar region, which was aggravated by rest but relieved by exercises. His red tongue with yellow, thin coating and thready pulse signified yang syndrome. Therefore, priority should be given to clearing away heat and removing dampness with due consideration to strengthening tendons and bones. Accordingly, the ZM bamboo cupping therapy was applied to his neck, shoulders, lower back and right hip to clear away heat and remove dampness, regulate the dragon and fire channels to relieve pain. In terms of the herbal medicinals, Rendongteng (Caulis Lonicerae Japonicae) is cold in nature. It is used as the sovereign drug due to its excellence at clearing away heat and regulating the dragon channel. Hujisheng (Herba Visci) and Duzhongteng (Cortex Parabarii) can remove dampness and dispel wind, strengthen tendons and bones, relieve pain and eliminate swelling. Shenjincao (Herba Lycopodii) is spicy and slightly bitter in taste and warm in nature. It can remove dampness and dispel wind and unblock the dragon channel. These three medicinals are used together as the minister drug. As the envoy drug, Liangmianzhen (Radix Zanthoxyli), which is spicy and bitter in taste and slightly warm in nature, can unblock the dragon and fire channels while Gancao (Radix et Rhizoma Glycyrrhizae) enables other herbal medicinals to better interact with each other. All the medicinals are used together to remove dampness and dispel wind, strengthen tendons and bones, relieve pain and eliminate swelling, resulting in synchronization of the heaven-qi, earth-qi and human-qi, smooth movement of qi and blood, and strong tendons and bones.

【病案三】

［Case 3］

李某，男，19 岁，2021 年 1 月 27 日初诊。

Patient: Li, a 19-year-old man; his first visit was on January 27, 2021.

主诉：腰骶、双下肢关节反复肿痛 9 年余，加重 3 个月。

Chief complaint:"I have had recurrent pain and swelling in my lumbosacral region and bilateral lower extremity joints for more than 9 years, which became worse 3 months ago."

现病史：患者 2011 年 8 月以右踝关节肿痛起病，逐渐出现右膝、右髋部疼痛，诊治不详，症状反复。2013 年 4 月在外院查 HLA-B27 阳性，ESR 39 mm/h，诊断为外周型脊柱关节病，随后来诊，诊断为幼年强直性脊柱炎。3 个月前患者出现左髋关节疼痛，随后出现右髋、腰骶部、胸背部、右足后跟明显疼痛，纳寐一般，二便调。舌质淡红，苔薄白，脉细。

History of present illness: The patient's disease started with pain and swelling in his right ankle in August 2011. Gradually, pain appeared in his right knee and hip. He could not report what treatment he had had. The symptoms were recurrent. In April 2013, he was diagnosed with peripheral spondyloarthropathy, based on his positive HLA-B27 test and ESR value of 39 mm/h at other hospital. Then, he sought medical care at our hospital, where he was diagnosed with juvenile AS. Three months ago, pain occurred in the joints of his left hip. Afterwards, he felt obvious pain in his right hip, lumbosacral region, chest, back and right heel. He reported good appetite, restful sleep, normal urination frequency and regular bowel movements. His tongue is reddish with white, thin coating. His pulse is thready.

目诊：勒答上龙脉脉络弯曲、有瘀点。甲诊：甲色淡红，半月痕暴露过少。壮医诊断：令扎－阴证－寒湿型。中医诊断：脊痹病－肾虚寒湿证。西医诊断：强直性脊柱炎。

Eye examination: The blood vessels of the eyes are curved with petechiae.

Nail examination: The nails are reddish with small fingernail lunulae.

Diagnosis in ZM:"Lingzha" characterized by cold-dampness syndrome, a type of yin syndrome.

Diagnosis in TCM: Kidney deficiency with cold-dampness syndrome, a type of spine impediment.

Diagnosis in WM: AS.

治疗：壮医药物竹罐疗法结合壮药内服治疗。

Treatment method: Apply the ZM bamboo cupping therapy and take Zhuang herbal medicinals.

处方如下。

Prescription.

（1）壮医药物竹罐疗法。部位：腰骶部 20 罐，隔 1 ～ 2 天 1 次，14 天为

1 个疗程。

(1) The ZM bamboo cupping therapy. Applied areas: Put 20 cups on the lumbosacral region, one time every 1~2 days, 14 days is a course of treatment.

（2）壮药内服。处方：牛大力 20 g，走马胎 15 g，五指毛桃 15 g，杜仲藤 10 g，伸筋草 15 g。5 剂，每日 1 剂，每剂水煎至 450 mL，分早中晚 3 次饭后温服。

(2) Zhuang herbal medicinals for oral administration. Prescription: Niudali (Radix Millettiae Speciosae) 20 g, Zoumatai (Radix et Rhizoma Ardisiae Gigantifoliae) 15 g, Wuzhimaotao (Radix Fici Hirtae) 15 g, Duzhongteng (Cortex Parabarii) 10 g and Shenjincao (Herba Lycopodii) 15 g. Decoct one dose of the medicinals with water to 450 mL daily and take the warm decoction 3 times a day after meals, 5 doses is a treatment course.

二诊（2021 年 2 月 2 日）：患者胸背部、腰骶部、双髋关节疼痛较前明显缓解，纳寐可，二便调，继服壮药内服方同前，以巩固疗效。

Second visit (on February 2, 2021): Pain in the joints of the patient's chest, back, lumbosacral region and hips was greatly relieved. He reported good appetite, restful sleep, normal urination frequency and regular bowel movements. Therefore, he was instructed to continue taking the same decoction to consolidate the efficacy.

按语：强直性脊柱炎常见于青年男性，属于壮医令扎范畴，缘于风毒、湿毒、寒毒侵袭，阻滞三道两路，使天、地、人三气不能同步而发本病。气血运行不畅，故关节疼痛。舌质红、苔白、脉沉为寒湿之征。故证属阴证，病位在脊柱、关节。

Summary statement: From the perspective of ZM, the patient's disease, AS which is often seen in young men, is a type of "Lingzha". Such type occurs due to the invasion of wind, dampness and cold, which blocks the three passages and two channels. The blockage will make the heaven-qi, earth-qi and human-qi unable to be synchronized, leading to the onset of the disease. Unsmooth movement of qi and blood leads to joint pain. Patients with such type of "Lingzha" usually have a red tongue with white coating and deep pulse, which are the signs of cold-dampness syndrome, a type of yin syndrome, and indicate that the disease sites are in the spine and joints.

本案治以祛风毒、散寒毒、壮筋骨为主。治疗多采用壮医药物竹罐疗法联合壮药内服的方法治疗。

Accordingly, the treatment should aim to dispel wind and dissipate cold, strengthen tendons and bones. The combination of the application of the ZM bamboo cupping therapy and oral administration of Zhuang herbal medicinals is preferable.

本案患者为青年男性，属强直性脊柱炎高发人群，病程长，症见胸背部、腰骶部、双髋关节疼痛。治宜以祛风毒、散寒毒、壮筋骨为主。采用壮医药物竹罐疗法施于腰骶部以疏通龙路火路、祛风湿、除湿毒、止痹痛。配合壮药内服，方中牛大力为性平味甘之品，能补气血，壮筋骨，祛湿解毒，活血，为主药。走马胎、杜仲藤祛风毒，除湿毒，通火路，消肿痛，合为帮药，共奏祛风毒、散寒毒、温经脉、壮筋骨之功。伸筋草味苦，性辛、温，能通调龙路火路，为带药。全方共奏祛风毒、散寒毒、止疼痛之效，使三气同步，气血运行通畅，筋骨得强。

As one of young men who have high prevalence of AS, the patient had long-term illness. The symptom was pain in the joints of his chest, back, lumbosacral region and hips. Therefore, the treatment aimed to dispel wind and dissipate cold, and strengthen tendons and bones. Accordingly, the ZM bamboo cupping therapy was applied to his lumbosacral region to unblock the dragon and fire channels, remove dampness and dispel wind, and eliminate arthralgia. In terms of the medicinals, Niudali (Radix Millettiae Speciosae) is sweet in taste and neutral in nature. It can tonify qi and blood, strengthen tendons and bones, remove dampness and toxins, activate blood, so it is used as the sovereign drug. As for the minister drug, Zoumatai (Radix et Rhizoma Ardisiae Gigantifoliae) and Duzhongteng (Cortex Parabarii) can remove dampness and dispel wind, unblock the fire channel, relieve pain and eliminate swelling. They can be used with the sovereign drug to dissipate cold and dispel wind, warm the meridians and collaterals, strengthen tendons and bones. As for the envoy drug, Shenjincao (Herba Lycopodii) is bitter and spicy in taste and warm in nature. It can unblock the dragon and fire channels. All the herbal medicinals are used together to remove dampness and dispel wind to relieve pain, resulting in synchronization of the heaven-qi, earth-qi and human-qi, smooth movement of qi and blood, and strong tendons and bones.

第二章　壮医药线点灸疗法
Chapter 2　Zhuang Medicine Medicated Thread Moxibustion

一、疗法概况
Ⅰ　Introduction

（一）发展历史
1　History of the Zhuang medicine medicated thread moxibustion

壮医药线点灸疗法由广西壮族自治区柳州市柳江区龙氏家族创立，是龙氏家族祖传的治病技法，主要在中国南方壮族地区流传，以广西柳江一带为轴心，辐射周边的壮族聚居地域。壮医药线点灸疗法起源于何时，目前仍没有发现确切的文字记载。有据可查的关于壮医药线点灸疗法的传承和应用历史，可追溯到 20 世纪 30 年代。当时龙氏家族已经开始用药线点灸疗法为当地乡亲治病，而且从 20 世纪 30 年代至 70 年代中后期，该疗法仅在龙氏家族内部口耳相传，药线的制作及操作技术等均未对外公开。壮医药线点灸疗法在龙氏家族中传承的大概过程如下：龙玉乾的曾祖父传给其儿媳妇龙覃氏，龙覃氏传给她的儿子龙见浤，龙见浤传给他的儿子龙玉乾。壮医药线点灸疗法传承到龙玉乾这一代时，龙玉乾打破家规，将疗法技术向世人公开。

The Zhuang medicine (ZM) medicated thread moxibustion therapy originates with an ancestor of a Long's family living in Liujiang County, Liuzhou City, Guangxi Zhuang Autonomous Region. It is popular in the settlements of the Zhuang nationality in South China, especially in Liujiang and its neighbouring Zhuang settlements. Although the start time of its application remains unknown due to lack of a clear written record, the existing documents show that its application can be traced back to the 1930s. At that time, the Long's family had been curing disease for many local people with this therapy such that it won a good reputation and public trust in the Lijiang River region. However, the theory and practice of this therapy, including medicated thread making and operating procedures, were only imparted within the Long's family by word of mouth, from Long Yuqian's parental great-grandfather, his parental grandmother to his father, Long Jianhong. Until the mid-1970s, Long Yuqian, the fourth generation successor, broke the family rules and made the therapy known to the public.

龙玉乾（1929—2006）是壮医药线点灸疗法的主要传人和实践应用推广者。在龙玉乾幼年时，父亲既向他传授医术，又不忘向他讲述龙氏家族的家传遗训："不求金玉重重富，但愿儿孙个个贤。"这是龙氏家族的祖训，也是龙氏家族的治家格言，更是龙氏家族的行医之道。龙玉乾自幼学习祖传壮医药线点灸疗法，并跟随祖母行医，积累了丰富的临床经验，此后，他又参加承钧中医班学习中医 4 年，将先辈传下来的壮医药线点灸疗法在实践中不断创新和发展。

As the main successor, Long Yuqian (1929—2006) played a leading role in popularizing the ZM medicated thread moxibustion. In his childhood, his father imparted the knowledge of the therapy and his family motto to him. The motto "Long's offspring is expected to be both virtuous and talented rather than wealthy" is also a maxim for family governance and the way of the Long's family practicing medicine. From childhood he was immersed in a setting which nurtured his appreciation of the therapy. He learned the therapy from his parental grandmother from an early age and accumulated much clinical experience. Afterwards, he studied TCM for 4 years by attending the Chengjun TCM class. He dedicated himself to the continuous innovation and development of the therapy.

1977 年上半年，龙玉乾被调到广西中医学院（现广西中医药大学）第一附属医院工作。他白天在门诊用壮医药线点灸疗法为患者治病，晚上和节假日的休息时间则进行药线点灸疗法教学。龙玉乾不仅将祖传经验和自己数十年所积累的实践经验和诊治体会传授给黄瑾明、黄汉儒等一大批医护工作者，还将祖传的药线点灸疗法进行了具体细致的整理，写成学习药线点灸疗法的讲稿一至五讲，共 10 万多字。

In the first half of 1977 when he was transferred to the First Affiliated Hospital of Guangxi College of Traditional Chinese Medicine (now Guangxi University of Chinese Medicine), Long Yuqian began to treat his patients with the ZM medicated thread moxibustion therapy in the outpatient department during the day while teaching the therapy in his spare time. He imparted the accumulated experience from his family and own medical practice to Huang Jinming, Huang Hanru and other medical practitioners. Also, he wrote up the therapy in 5 manuscripts of over 10, 000 words in total.

20 世纪 80 年代末，龙玉乾回到家乡柳州。他不仅继续出诊治病，而且继续带徒办班，传承星火。工作之余，他刻苦钻研民族医药，勤于笔耕，结合丰富的临床实践经验著书立说，或是编撰教材，或是将自己的治疗心得撰写成多篇论文在民族医药大会上进行交流。

In the late 1980s, after going back to his hometown, Liuzhou, Long Yuqian continued to cure disease for people and continued education course for training practitioners of the therapy. In his spare time, he delved into ethnic medicine and put his thoughts into words. Subsequently, he compiled these thoughts and his own experience of medical practice into teaching materials. Also, his experience was published in the form of academic essays for academic communication at ethnic medicine conferences.

黄瑾明率先开展对壮医药线点灸疗法的发掘整理、研究提高及推广应用，并于 1985 年 4 月创建广西第一家壮医门诊部——广西中医学院壮医门诊部，把壮医药线点灸疗法这一壮族民间的治病技法首次引进高等医药院校，并在与班秀文、黄汉儒、黄鼎坚等人的倾力合作下对壮医药线点灸疗法进行深入地挖掘整理研究及推广应用。

As a pioneer in studying, improving and popularizing the ZM medicated thread moxibustion therapy, Huang Jinming first introduced the folk treatment technique into a medical institution of higher education by setting up the ZM clinic of Guangxi College of Traditional Chinese Medicine in April 1985. He also cooperated with Ban Xiuwen, Huang Hanru and Huang Dingjian to further study, improve and popularize the therapy.

1986 年 1 月，在龙玉乾的指导下，黄瑾明等人将龙玉乾祖传的药线点灸技术、临床经验及壮医门诊部应用药线点灸疗法治疗疾病积累的临床资料等进行全面分析和系统整理，初步总结、归纳、提炼出药线点灸疗法的壮医指导理论、点灸选穴原则、用穴规律、操作技术及临床应用规律等内容，编写成《壮医药线点灸疗法》一书。《壮医药线点灸疗法》是壮医发展史上第一部以"壮医"命名的著作，荣获广西优秀科普作品二等奖。此外，由黄瑾明主持完成的"壮医药线点灸疗法的发掘整理及疗效验证研究"项目，荣获国家中医药科技进步奖二等奖和广西医药卫生科技进步奖一等奖，为壮医发展史上首项科研成果；"壮医药线点灸疗法的研究和教学实践研究"项目，首次把壮医的科研成果转化成教材，并率先在大学本科教学中开设壮医药线点灸疗法的课程，获广西优秀教学成果奖二等奖。

In January 1986, the book *The Zhuang Medicine Medicated Thread Moxibustion* was published. It contains guiding theories, principles of acupoints selection, operating procedures and application rules of the therapy, which were derived from Long Yuqian's, Huang Jinming's and other co-workers' thorough analysis, sorting, preliminary summarization, induction and distilling of the cumulative experience of the therapy from the Long's family and from the ZM clinic. As the first book named after ZM, it won the second prize of Guangxi Best Popular Science Works. As the first research accomplishment, the research program *The Exploration, Collation and Efficacy Verification of the Zhuang Medicine Medicated Thread Moxibustion* that was presided over by Huang Jinming won the second prize of state Scientific and Technological Progress of Traditional Chinese Medicine Award and the first prize of Guangxi Scientific and Technological Progress of Medicine and Health Award. The research results from Huang Jinming's program *The Research on the Zhuang Medicine Medicated Thread Moxibustion and Its Teaching Practice* were transformed into teaching materials which were used in the undergraduate course of The ZM Medicated Thread Moxibustion at university. The program won the second prize of Guangxi Outstanding Teaching Achievements Award.

接着，黄瑾明等人又依据龙氏临床经验及壮医门诊部积累的病例治疗资料，提炼出精华部分，整理出版了一部临床应用专著《壮医药线点灸临床治验录》，并拍摄出版了《壮医药线点灸疗法》电视教学录像片（中英文版）。在国内及美国、英国、澳大利亚、新加坡等国家推广应用，取得了较好的社会效益。

Afterwards, based on their previous research accomplishments, Huang Jinming and his co-workers published a monograph dedicated to clinical practice of the therapy, *Record of the Treatment Experience of the Zhuang Medicine Medicated Thread Moxibustion*. Also the education video, *The Zhuang Medicine Medicated Thread Moxibustion*, was produced and promoted in China and other countries such as the USA, the UK, Australia and Singapore, bearing much fruit.

班秀文、黄瑾明等先行者，根据龙玉乾祖传经验，从讲座、大学生兴趣小组开始，向大学生传播壮医药线点灸疗法。尤其是黄瑾明，率先在大学本科教学中开设壮医药线点灸疗法的课程，并把自己主持完成的"壮医药线点灸疗法的研究和教学实践研究"项目成果充实到教材中，使药线点灸疗法这一壮族民间的治病技法首度被引进国家的医疗、科研、教学单位，并广泛应用于临床各科，使壮医药线点灸疗法得到更好的传承和发展。2000 年开始，广西中医学院将壮医药线点灸疗法的授课对象从原有的中医学专业学生扩大到全校所有的医科专业学生。由黄瑾明、林辰编写出版的壮医学专业本科系列教材之一《壮医药线点灸学》于 2006 年出版。该教材明确了壮医药线点灸疗法以阴阳为本、天地人三气同步论、三道两路学说及气血均衡论等为指导理论，规范了临床用穴选穴及操作技术。广西中医学院将壮医药线点灸学设为壮医本科的专业必修课，并设为其他各专业的选修课，从而规范了壮医药线点灸学的教育，加大了壮医药线点灸人才的培养力度，为壮医药线点灸疗法的传承、发展、创新奠定了良好的基础。2008 年，壮医药线点灸学被评为广西中医学院校级精品课程。2009年，壮医药线点灸学被评为广西壮族自治区级精品课程。2011 年，壮医药线点灸疗法入选第三批国家级非物质文化遗产名录。2012 年，"壮医药线点灸学"获得特色专业及一体化课程建设项目立项。

Ban Xiuwen, Huang Jinming and other forerunners introduced the ZM medicated thread moxibustion to college students by delivering lectures and starting interest groups. In particular, with the efforts of Huang Jinming who transformed the research results from his program *The Research on the Zhuang Medicine Medicated Thread Moxibustion and Its Teaching Practice* into the teaching materials used in the undergraduate course, the therapy was first introduced into China's medical, scientific research and education institutions and began to be applied to multiple clinical departments, thereby being better inherited and developed. Since the year 2000, the therapy has been taught to students from other majors in addition to students from TCM majors at Guangxi College of Traditional Chinese Medicine. As one of the textbook series for the undergraduate program in ZM, *The Zhuang Medicine Medicated Thread Moxibustion*, which is compiled by Huang Jinming and Lin Chen and published in 2006, specifies guiding theories of the therapy, including the yin-yang theory, the thought of synchronization of the heaven-qi, earth-qi and human-qi, the theory of three passages and two channels and the thought of harmony of qi and blood. It also provides specifications for acupoints selection and operation. The ZM medicated thread moxibustion has become a required course for ZM majors and an optional course for other medical majors at Guangxi University of Chinese Medicine. This standardizes the education of the therapy and helps produce its practitioners who in turn make contributions to the inheritance, development and innovation of the therapy. In 2008, the course was rated as a university-level quality course and in 2009 as a provincial-level quality course. In 2011, the therapy was inscribed on the Representative List of State-level Intangible Cultural Heritage of Humanity. In 2012, the course became one of the projects for construction of characteristic specialties and integrated curricula.

壮医药线点灸疗法不仅在教学方面获得了蓬勃发展，在基础与应用研究方面也得到前所未有的发展，焕发出勃勃生机。许多医务工作者、学者采用现代科学技术方法和手段，对药线点灸疗法进行临床疗效观察及技术操作规范与应用的研究，不断拓展其适应证，筛选其优势病种，并对壮医药线点灸疗法的作用机制进行实验研究，以揭示药线点灸疗法的基本作用。对壮医药线点灸疗法基础和应用的深入研究取得了令人瞩目的成果，壮医药线点灸学理论体系内容得到不断充实和完善，随着理论层面得到不断的梳理、总结、凝练和提升，临床应用规范也得到不断完善，壮医药线点灸疗法临床服务可及性将会不断提高、医疗与预防保健服务能力不断增强。

To date, the ZM medicated thread moxibustion has vigorously developed in terms of education and research on its basic theories and application. By means of the methodologies of science and technology, many medical practitioners and scholars have made determined efforts to expand the indications of the therapy and investigate what diseases it has remarkable efficacy on by observing its clinical curative effectiveness and studying its technical operating specifications and application. Experimental research on its mechanism of action has also been conducted to reveal its fundamental functions. The in-depth research on the therapy has born much fruit. This has enabled its theories to be constantly enriched and technical operating specifications to be continuously improved, resulting in its higher accessibility and growing capacity in medical and preventive care services.

（二）治疗机理

2　Treatment mechanism

壮医学认为，疾病的产生是各种邪毒如痧、瘴、蛊、毒、风、湿等，通过龙路、火路在人体体表形成的网结侵犯人体，正邪相争，使天、地、人三气不能同步，脏腑骨肉功能失调，气血紊乱及三道两路受阻所致；或人体正虚，天、地、人三气不能同步，脏腑、气血、骨肉、三道两路功能减退，产生水毒、痰毒、食毒及瘀毒等滞留体内，使三道两路受阻，气血运行不畅所致。

From the perspective of ZM, diseases are caused by the failure of synchronization of the heaven-qi, earth-qi and human-qi, dysfunction of zang-fu organs, muscles and bones, disharmony of qi and blood and/or blockage of the three passages and two channels. These pathological changes occur when pathogenic toxins, including filth, miasma, parasite, wind and/or dampness, invade the human body and cause struggle between healthy qi and pathogenic factors. These pathological changes can also be caused by retention of toxins such as water, phlegm, food, blood stasis. These toxins emerge in the body due to the deficiency of the healthy qi, failure of synchronization of the heaven-qi, earth-qi and human-qi or decline in the function of zang-fu organs, qi, blood, muscles and bones.

龙路、火路内属脏腑，外络肢节，贯通上下左右，将内部的脏腑同外部的各种组织及器官联结成一个有机的整体。龙路、火路在人体体表形成的网结（穴位）是脏腑气血骨肉之外延，是人体气血的出入之处，也是邪毒的出入之处，在体表肌肤上表现为压痛、胀、麻等反应，是药线点灸疗法施灸的主要部位。

As part of zang-fu organs, the dragon and fire channels are the meridians and collaterals running through the whole body to make tissues and other organs connected to be an organic whole. The points (i.e. acupoints) where the dragon and fire channels intersect on the superficies of the body are the places through which zang-fu organs, qi, blood, muscles and bones perceive the environment. They are also the places where qi, blood and pathogenic toxins enter and exit. Pain, feeling of swelling and numbness occur when they are pressed, so they are the areas where the ZM medicated thread moxibustion is applied.

壮医药线点灸疗法的治病机理，是以其温热、药效及对人体网结（穴位）的刺激，通过龙路、火路传导，鼓舞人体正气，祛毒外出，恢复天、地、人三气同步，正常发挥脏腑、骨肉、气血的功能，平衡气血，畅通三道两路，使人体各部功能恢复正常，从而促使疾病好转或痊愈。

When the therapy is applied, Zhuang medicine enters the body via stimulated and warmed acupoints and runs along the dragon and fire channels to replenish the healthy qi and draw out toxins, resulting in restoration of synchronization of the heaven-qi, earth-qi and human-qi, recovery of the function of zang-fu organs, muscles and bones, harmony of qi and blood, and smooth the three passages and two channels. Consequently, diseases will improve or be cured.

（三）主要功效
3　Main efficacy

根据临床实践总结和实验研究结果，整理出壮医药线点灸疗法具有以下主要功效。

Experience from clinical practice and results from experimental research show the following efficacy of the ZM medicated thread moxibustion.

1. 祛风毒、湿毒、寒毒

3.1　To remove wind, dampness and cold

风毒、湿毒、寒毒通过龙路、火路在人体体表形成的网结（穴位）入侵人体而致病，或因机体脏腑、气血、骨肉、三道两路功能减退，使风毒、湿毒、寒毒内生而致病。壮医药线点灸疗法具有较好的祛风毒、湿毒、寒毒的作用，在临床上用于治疗皮肤瘙痒、荨麻疹、稻田皮炎、湿疹、脚气病、腰腿疼痛、感冒、头痛、胃脘痛、腹痛等由风毒、湿毒、寒毒引起的疾病，均可取得显著的疗效。

Diseases are caused by invasion of wind, dampness and/or cold through acupoints along the dragon and fire channels or internal emergence of these toxins when the functions of zang-fu organs, qi, blood, muscles, bones, three passages and two channels are in decline. Since the therapy is excellent at removing these toxins, it is used to treat the diseases caused by these toxins, including skin itching, urticaria, rice field dermatitis, eczema, beriberi, lumbago and leg pain, cold, headache, epigastric pain, abdominal pain.

2. 祛痧毒、瘴毒、热毒

3.2　To remove filth, miasma and heat

痧毒、瘴毒、热毒是导致机体发病的常见因素。痧毒、瘴毒、热毒滞留人体后可引发多种病变，如恶寒发热、头晕胀痛、恶心呕吐、腹痛腹泻、全身肌肉酸痛、口腔溃疡、咽喉发炎肿痛、痔疮发炎肿痛、疮疔红肿疼痛等。壮医药线点灸疗法具有较好的祛痧毒、瘴毒、热毒的作用，可用于治疗痧毒、瘴毒及热毒所引起的多种病证。

As common pathogenic factors, internal retention of filth, miasma and/or heat can cause many diseases, including fever with chills, headache with dizziness, nausea, diarrhea with abdominal pain, muscle soreness, mouth ulcer, inflammation, swelling and pain of throat and hemorrhoids and redness, swelling and pain of furuncle. Since the therapy is excellent at removing filth, miasma and heat, it is used to treat the diseases caused by filth, miasma and heat.

3. 祛水毒、痰毒、食毒

3.3　To remove the retention of water, phlegm and food

水毒、痰毒、食毒是常见的内生毒邪。当机体脏腑、气血、骨肉、三道两路功能减退，可产生水毒、痰毒、食毒滞留体内而致病。壮医药线点灸疗法具有较好的通调水道、气道、谷道的作用，在临床上可用于治疗水毒引起的胸胁积水、下肢水肿、腹水、小便不利等，或痰毒引起的痰多、咳嗽、咳喘等，或痰毒闭阻火路引起的肌肤麻木不仁、麻痹、偏瘫、视物不清等，或食毒引起的消化不良、恶心、呕吐、胃胀痛、腹胀痛、腹泻、便秘等病证。

Retention of water, phlegm and food is prone to emerge in the body when the functions of zang-fu organs, qi, blood, muscles, bones, three passages and two channels are in decline. Internal retention of water, phlegm and food will lead to diseases. For example, retention of water may lead to pleural effusion, lower extremity edema, ascites and dysuria. Retention of phlegm can lead to profuse sputum, cough and cough with wheezing, and block the fire channel. The blockage may result in skin numbness, paralysis, hemiplegia and blurred vision. Diseases caused by food toxin include indigestion, nausea, vomiting, stomachache, abdominal pain, diarrhea and constipation. The therapy is excellent at regulating the water, qi and grain passages, so it can be used to treat the diseases mentioned above.

4. 祛瘀通路

3.4　To remove blood stasis and unblock the passages and channels

壮医药线点灸疗法用于各种血证，既有活血祛瘀的作用，又有止血的效果。一般来说，点灸具有活血作用的穴位可以祛除瘀血，点灸具有止血作用的穴位可以控制出血。然而祛瘀和止血两者是互相关联的，若属于瘀血导致的出血症，只有先祛瘀后才能止血。此外，还有一些既有活血作用又有止血作用的穴位，具有双向调节作用，关键在于认真辨清病因病性，精心选好穴位。

The therapy can be used for many blood syndromes since it can activate blood, remove blood stasis and stop bleeding. Specifically, it is applied to acupoints with the effect of activating blood to remove blood stasis and to those with hemostatic effect to stop bleeding. Since the removal of blood stasis and hemostasis are correlated, for hemorrhagic disease caused by blood stasis, the removal of blood stasis should be prior to hemostasis. In terms of acupoints with the effect of activating blood and stopping bleeding, either the removal of blood stasis or hemostasis is performed in the first place as appropriate. Therefore, identification of the etiology of a disease should be prior to the selection of acupoints.

5. 调气安神

3.5　To adjust qi to tranquilize the mind

壮医药线点灸疗法可调和气血，调节人体阴阳的偏盛偏衰，使机体恢复气血协调、阴阳平衡、精神安宁的状态。壮医药线点灸疗法用于治疗一些情绪不宁的疾病，如失眠、紧张、焦虑、神经官能症、更年期综合征等均有一定的效果。

The therapy can be used to harmonize qi and blood and neutralize abnormal exuberance and debilitation of yin or yang to restore qi and blood balance, harmonize yin and yang and tranquilize the mind. Accordingly, it can treat the diseases caused by emotional disorders, including insomnia, anxiety, depression, neurosis and menopausal syndrome.

6. 补虚强体

3.6　To reinforce deficiency to strengthen the body

选择有强壮补益作用的穴位定期进行壮医药线点灸治疗，可以起到鼓舞人体正气、增强体质、防病保健的作用。

The regular application of the therapy to acupoints with the effect of reinforcing deficiency can tonify the healthy qi, strengthen the body, prevent diseases and protect health.

二、技法特色
Ⅱ　Characteristics of the therapy

（一）理论特色
1　Theoretical features

1. 阴阳为本论
1.1　The yin-yang theory

壮医阴阳为本的概念最早由黄汉儒在《壮医理论体系概述》一文中提出。黄汉儒认为，阴阳为本是壮医的天人自然观，"大自然的各种变化，壮医学认为都是阴阳对立、阴阳互根、阴阳消长、阴阳平衡、阴阳转化的反映和结果"。阴阳为本是"阴阳为本源""阴阳为根本"之意，阴阳的存在及运动变化是天地万物运动变化的本源，阴阳的运动变化是天地万物中普遍存在的一种客观现象。根据壮医阴阳为本理论，人体生理病理的各种变化、各种药物及治疗技法所起的作用、疾病的转归等都是人体内部阴阳运动变化的结果。健康是阴阳双方协调平衡的结果。

The concept of yin and yang being fundamental principles in the universe in ZM was first described in Huang Hanru's *An Overview of the Theoretical System of Zhuang Medicine*. According to Huang, it is a philosophical concept about human and nature in ZM. It is widely applied to ZM that changes in nature result from opposition, mutual rooting, waxing and waning, balance and conversion of yin and yang. The ceaseless motion of both yin and yang which are opposing and complementing each other—an objective phenomenon, gives rise to all changes seen in the world. Accordingly, the motion of yin and yang of the human body results in physiological and pathological changes in the human body, curative effects of drugs and treatment techniques, and conversion of diseases. Yin-yang harmony guarantees health.

2. 三气同步论

1.2　The theory of synchronization of the heaven-qi, earth-qi and human-qi

壮医天、地、人三气同步的概念最早由老壮医覃保霖总结出来，经过对民间壮医进行实地调查，证实确有此说，是根据壮语"人不得逆天地"或"人必须顺天地"意译而来。天指天气，地指地气，两者合称天地自然之气；人，即人生命的活动规律。天在上，其气以降为顺，主降；地在下，其气以升为要，主升；人在中，其气以纳为宜，主和。天、地、人三气都处在不断地运动变化之中，并且相互影响，相互作用。天、地、人三气同步是指天、地、人三部之气协调平稳运行，才能保持人体最佳生命状态，即人体要保持健康的生理状态，不仅自身各部的生理功能需协调一致，而且人体必须与外界环境保持协调同步的关系。天、地、人三气同步论不仅强调人自身的整体性，也强调人与自然界的协调统一性。天气主降，地气主升，天地之气上下交流感应，互为因果，导致万物的生长化收藏。人类作为自然界的产物和重要组成部分，必然受自然规律的支配和制约，天地之气不断运动和变化会直接或间接地影响人体。天地之气对人的影响主要表现如下：其一，不仅人（人类）是天地之气的产物，而且每个人（自然人）的孕育也需要天地之气的滋养，天地之气不足会引起人先天的不足，甚至夭亡；其二，人出生以后的生长壮老已的生命历程，都受到天地之气的影响和制约，人要健康长寿必须顺应自然界天地之气的变化。壮医学认为，天、地、人三气同步是以天、地为主导的三者之间的"同步"状态。"同步"是指三者之间协调平衡的一种状态，是常态。天、地、人三气同步的核心就是一个"动"字，即宇宙天地永远处在不断运动变化之中，人随着天地之气的运动变化而变化。人对天地之气的变化要主动适应，才能维持生存和健康的常度。如不能适应，就会产生疾病。

The concept of synchronization of the heaven-qi, earth-qi and human-qi was first presented by the ZM practitioner, Qin Baolin, who paraphrased the old saying "human beings have to obey nature" in the Zhuang nationality after conducting field investigations. The heaven-qi and earth-qi exist in nature while the human-qi maintains life activities. The heaven is high above the earth, so the heaven-qi is desired to descend while the earth-qi desired to ascend. For human beings who exist between the heaven and the earth, qi reception is desired. These three kinds of qi constantly move and change and interact with each other. Their synchronization, which is dominated by the heaven-qi and earth-qi, refers to harmony of them and thus human body maintains in good condition. In other words, to maintain health, the human body has to coordinate the physiological functions of its organs and be in adaptive conformity with the variations of the natural environment. The theory of synchronization of the heaven-qi, earth-qi and human-qi emphasizes the integrity of the human body itself and the harmony between the body and nature. The interaction of the heaven-qi and earth-qi enables all living things to grow ups and downs. As a product and an important component of nature, human beings are bound to be governed and constrained by natural laws and influenced, directly or indirectly, by the interaction between the heaven-qi and earth-qi. The manifestations of influences of the heaven-qi and earth-qi on human beings include: a) Human beings are the product of the heaven-qi and earth-qi. In the process of gestating lives, these two kinds of qi are required. The inadequacy of them can lead to birth defects and even fetal or child mortality; and b) human life development is governed and constrained by the heaven-qi and earth-qi. The realization of longevity requires the body to be in adaptive conformity with the variations of the heaven-qi and earth-qi.

3. 三道两路论

1.3　The theory of three passages and two channels

三道，即谷道、气道、水道，是维持人体生命活动所需营养物质化生、贮藏、输布、运行的场所。分而言之，谷道是食物消化吸收和精微输布之通道；气道是人体一身之气化生、输布之处所；水道则是人体水液化生、贮藏、输布、运行的地方。五谷禀天地之气以生长，赖天地之气以收藏，得天地之气以滋养人体，其进入人体得以消化吸收之通道即称为谷道，主要是指食道和胃肠。水为生命之源，人体通过水道进水出水，与大自然发生直接、密切的联系。水道与谷道同源而分流，在吸取水谷精微营养物质后，谷道排出粪便，水道主要排出汗、尿。水道的调节枢纽为肾与膀胱。气道是人体之气与大自然之气相互交换的通道，主要进出口为口鼻，交换枢纽为肺。三道畅通，调节有度，人体之气就能与天地之气保持同步协调平衡，人体即处于健康状态。龙路与火路是壮医对人体内虽未直接与大自然相通，但却是维持人体生理功能和反映疾病动态的两条极为重要的内在封闭通路的命名。壮族传统认为龙是制水的，龙路即人体内血液的通道，其功能主要是为内脏骨肉传输营养。龙路有干线，有网络，遍布全身，循环往来，其中枢在心脏。火为触发之物，其性迅速，感之灼热。壮医学认为，火路为人体内传感之道，用现代语言来说也可称为"信息通道"，其中枢在巧坞（脑）。火路同龙路一样，有干线，有网络，遍布全身，使正常人体能在极短时间内感受外界的各种信息和刺激，并经中枢巧坞的处理，迅速做出反应，以此来适应外界的各种变化，实现三气同步的生理平衡。

The three passages refer to the grain passage, qi passage and water passage, where nutrients required for the maintenance of human life activities are produced, stored, transported and transformed. Specifically, the grain passage is the place where food is digested and absorbed, from which refined essence is derived and transported to the whole body; the qi passage is the place for production and transportation of qi; and in the water passage, water is produced, stored, transported and transformed. Crops grow up and down and contain nourishing substances essential to the human body by the qi of heaven and earth. The grain passage refers to the esophagus and gastrointestinal tract. As the source of all living things, water enters and leaves the body via the water passage. It has a direct and close relationship with nature. Food essence is produced and transformed in the water and grain passages, but waste substance is discharged as feces through the grain passage while excessive water discharged as sweat and urine through the water passage where the kidney and bladder play the leading role. Qi enters and exits the body through the mouth and nose. Exchange of qi from nature and that in the body takes place in the qi passage, of which the hub for qi exchange is the lung. Smooth three passages and good coordination among them can synchronize the human-qi with the heaven-qi and earth-qi, thereby maintaining human health. In terms of the dragon and fire channels, although they are not directly connected with nature, they are two extremely important closed channels that maintain physiological functions and reflect diseases. According to the traditional cognition of the Zhuang nationality, the dragon produces water, so in ZM, the dragon channel refers to blood vessels transporting nutrients to zang-fu organs, bones and muscles. The dragon channel whose center is the heart consists of main and branch lines which are all over the body and form a cycle. As a trigger, fire develops fast and produces heat, so in ZM, the fire channel whose center is brain ("Qiaowu" in the Zhuang language) functions like a sensor reacting to the environment. It can also be called "information channel" in modern language. As with the dragon channel, the fire channel have main and branch lines which enable the body to immediately sense the information and stimuli from the environment, and then quickly respond after the processing of the brain. Thus, the body can keep in adaption to the variations of the environment, resulting in physiological balance of synchronization of three kinds of qi.

（二）临床特色

2　Clinical features

壮医药线点灸疗法具有以下 5 个方面的显著特点。

There are five notable features as follows:

（1）适应证范围广。壮医药线点灸疗法可以治疗内科、外科、皮肤科、妇产科、小儿科、眼科、口腔科、耳鼻喉科等涉及的常见病、多发病及一些疑难杂症。

(1) A wide range of indications: The ZM medicated thread moxibustion can treat common and intractable diseases of internal medicine, surgery, dermatology, gynecology, pediatrics, ophthalmology, stomatology, and ENT[*].

（2）优势病种突出。壮医药线点灸疗法对一些疾病疗效非常好，如感冒发烧、红眼病、偏头痛、痛经及接触性皮炎等。

(2) Remarkable efficacy on some diseases: The therapy has remarkable efficacy on some diseases, including cold with fever, red-eyed disease, migraine, dysmenorrhea and contact dermatitis.

（3）简、便、廉、验、捷。壮医药线点灸疗法所需设备简单，有灯火（或火柴、蜡烛、打火机）和药线即可施灸治病。药线成本低，可以随身携带，施灸不受场所限制，随时随地均可以治疗。

(3) Simplicity, convenience and quickness in operation, low material consumption cost, and effectiveness. The application of the therapy demands simple devices, namely, a match, lit candle or lighter, and low-cost medicated threads. These devices are portable so the therapy can be applied anywhere and anytime.

（4）无毒副作用，无污染。药线点灸时局部仅有蚁咬样灼热感，无难忍之痛苦；点灸后无疤痕，无后遗症，没有任何毒副作用，安全可靠。药线点燃后无烟雾形成，燃后烟灰俱灭，无环境污染。

(4) Be free from toxic and side effect and environmental pollution: There is merely an ant-bite-like burning sensation in applied areas, which is tolerable. The moxibustion does not cause scars, complications or toxic and side effect. Medicated threads are environmentally friendly because they burn without giving off smoke and turn to ash.

（5）协调治疗作用。壮医药线点灸疗法可以单独应用，也可以与其他疗法（包括内治法和外治法）联合应用。壮医药线点灸疗法与其他方法联合应用时，不影响其他疗法的疗效，并且可起到疗效协同作用，可提高综合治疗的效果。

---

* ENT stands for ear, nose and throat.

(5) Compatibility: The therapy can be applied alone or in combination with other internal or external therapies. It will not affect the efficacy of other therapies. Instead, the therapies can work together to enhance curative effects.

（三）选穴特色

3　Features of acupoints selection

1. 以环为穴

3.1　Acupoints around the affected area

以环为穴是指可根据疾病的病因病机选用具有相应主治功效的环穴作为治疗用穴。

Select acupoints around the affected area according to the cause and mechanism of the disease.

2. 以应为穴

3.2　Reaction points

以应为穴是指疾病在人体体表某一部位有反应点，在这处反应点取一组穴位进行治疗的取穴方法。以应为穴的取穴方法又可以分为左右对称取穴法和上下对称取穴法。

"Reaction points" means to select points on the body surface, which reflect the disease. The selection method includes right-left point combination and upper-lower point combination.

（1）左右对称取穴法。以脊柱为中线，将人体分为左右两部分，这两部分相互对称，形态和结构均极为相似。且这两部分的生理功能相似，故其病理反应也相似，可以互为反射区。如两手、两肘、两侧臂膀、两肩、两肋、两侧下肢等，如果一侧发生病痛，在另一侧的相同部位就会出现反应点，按压反应点患者就会有不同程度的疼痛感或酸胀感；临床上可在反应点取穴进行治疗。

(1) Right-left point combination: The spine divides the body vertically into equal right and left halves, of which the shape, structure and physiological functions are similar, so their pathological reactions are similar. Since these two sides are each other's reflection area, if there is a disease site on one side of the body, for example, on one of the arms, shoulders, ribs, lower extremities, reaction points will appear

at the same location on its corresponding opposite side. Patients may feel pain or soreness with varying degrees. It is feasible to select reaction points as acupoints for treatment in clinical practice.

（2）上下对称取穴法。人体的上下两部分在临床上基本遵循形态、结构、生理功能上相似度较大的原则，故其病理反应也相似，可以互为反射区，进行取穴点灸治疗，例如上肢和下肢、肩关节和髋关节等。具体取穴方法如下：医者用自己的手掌及手指指腹，根据患者的疾病情况，分别对患者天、地、人三部体表的上下、左右相关对应点进行触摸，寻找相应的穴位或治疗点。如触摸到局部有硬结、压痛感、酸胀感或舒适感等的反应点，则这个点就是疾病的体表反应穴，即可以在此处取穴进行治疗。

(2) Upper-lower point combination: From the clinical perspective, the shape, structure and physiological functions of the upper- and lower-body sessions are similar, so their pathological reactions are similar. They can be considered as each other's reflection area for acupoints selection. For example, the upper limb is paired with the lower limb while the shoulder joints are paired with the hip joints. According to the patient's medical conditions, the practitioner feels the affected area in an up-to-down and left-to-right motion with their palm and finger pulp to look for reactions points at which there are subcutaneous induration, tenderness, soreness, and/or sensation of sensitivity or comfort. Then, the therapy is applied to these points.

3. 以痛为穴

3.3　Ashi acupoints

以痛为穴是指通过循切、按压找到压痛点及疾病在人体体表的相应反应点，无论是局部还是远端，都可以在疼痛的部位或相应压痛点的位置，选取一个或多个甚至一组穴位作为治疗用穴。

"Ashi acupoints" means to find the points by eliciting tenderness at the disease site and in the corresponding area far from the disease site. Then, select one or more points for treatment.

壮医学认为，用以痛为穴的治疗原则所取的穴位，实质上位于人体壮气游行出入之处，也恰恰是正邪相交、激烈斗争之处，因此按以痛为穴原则所取的穴位能收到较好的临床疗效。

From the perspective of ZM, Ashi acupoints are the places where the healthy qi and pathogenic qi struggle, so remarkable efficacy can be obtained by using these points.

4. 以灶为穴

3.4　Acupoints at the disease site

气血运行受阻，滞而为瘀，瘀积为灶。灶即为肿、胀或痛。以灶为穴是指在病灶部位选取一个或多个甚至一组穴位作为施治穴位。

Unsmooth movement of qi and blood can lead to qi stagnation and blood stasis, which causes an area of the body to be diseased. Such area is characterized by swelling, soreness or pain. Accordingly, select one or more points at the diseased area for treatment.

5. 以边为穴

3.5　Acupoints along the edge

以边为穴是指以人体的肌肉边、肌腱边、骨边为标志点，通过摸、捏或按、压的方法，选取一个或多个甚至一组穴位作为施治穴位。

Feel, pinch and press the edge of muscles, tendons and skeletal muscles to look for acupoints. Then, select one or more points for treatment.

6. 以间为穴

3.6　Acupoints in depressions

以间为穴是指在肌体的肌肉之间、肌腱之间、骨之间的孔隙或凹陷处取穴以治疗疾病。

Select points between two muscles, two tendons and two bones for treatment.

7. 以验为穴

3.7　Acupoints selection based on experience

以验为穴是指以壮医在长期临床实践中积累总结并流传下来的特定的穴位或穴位组，即壮医经验穴，作为施治穴位。

Based on the cumulative experience of ZM practitioners in long-term medical practice, there are individual and paired acupoints uniquely used in ZM acupuncture and moxibustion.

8. 龙氏取穴原则

3.8　Principle of acupoints selection from the Long's family

龙氏取穴原则即"寒手热背肿在梅，痿肌痛沿麻络央，唯有痒疾抓长子，各疾施灸不离乡"的取穴原则。"寒手"指有畏寒发冷症状者，以选取手部穴位为主；"热背"指发热体温升高者，以选取背部穴位为主；"肿在梅"指有肿块或皮损类疾病者，在肿块或皮损边缘及中央选取一组约 5 个呈梅花形分布的穴位，在临证时应根据肿块的大小决定其周边所点灸的穴位为 4 个、6 个、8 个或更多，不必拘泥于点灸 5 个穴，也不必固定在某个位置上，应根据病情的需要而改变；"痿肌"指肌肉萎缩者，在该萎缩肌肉上选取主要穴位；"麻络央"指麻木不仁者，选取其患病部位一段经络的中央点为主要穴位；"抓长子"指由皮疹类疾病引起皮肤瘙痒者，选取首先出现的疹子或最大的疹子为主要穴位。

According to the cumulative experience that is imparted from one generation of the Long's family to another, the medicated thread moxibustion is applied to acupoints on the local and/or adjacent areas of the disease site for treatment. Specifically, select points on the hands to treat those with intolerance of cold and chills. Select points on the back for those with a fever. To treat bumps or skin lesions, normally, use four specific points along the edge of a bump or lesion and one point in its center. These five points are distributed in the shape of a plum flower. However, possibly take six, eight or more points along the edge due to the different conditions of the disease. Besides, take points on non-fixed areas as appropriate. Take points in the atrophied muscle as the primary ones to treat muscle atrophy. Select points in the middle of the meridian in the numb area as the primary ones to treat numbness. And for the treatment of skin itching due to rash-type diseases, select points on the area as the primary ones where rashes first appeared or the largest rash is.

此外，还可以根据病情需要，按照中医经络腧穴的主治功效选取适当的中医腧穴作为药线点灸用穴。

In addition, according to the conditions of the disease, points along the affected meridian/channel, which are normally taken in TCM, can be selected as appropriate for the medicated thread moxibustion.

三、操作规范

Ⅲ Specifications for operation

（一）前期准备

1 Pre-treatment preparation

进行药线点灸前，首先要做好以下 5 个方面的准备工作。

Prepare for the application of the ZM medicated thread moxibustion as follows.

（1）备好火源。使用酒精灯、蜡烛、煤油灯等均可，但不宜使用含有有毒物质的火源如蚊香等。

(1) Fire source: Prepare a fire source, such as an alcohol lamp, candle or kerosene lamp. Do not use the substances that contain poisons, for example, mosquito coils.

（2）备好药线。药线成批购回后可以用深色的瓶子或深色的塑料袋密封存放，宜放在阴暗干燥处，不宜放在高温或靠近火炉的地方，也不宜让阳光照射，不宜频繁打开瓶盖，以免损失药效。药线准备遵照"用多少准备多少"的原则。

(2) Medicated threads: Put medicated threads in dark sealed storage containers or plastic bags. Put medicated threads purchased in bulk in a dark and dry place instead of a place with high temperature or near a stove. Do not frequently open the containers or bags to prevent the loss of efficacy. Follow the principle of "preparing medicated threads in right amounts".

（3）选好体位。一般宜让患者选用坐位或卧位，使施灸穴位充分显露，力求患者舒适，避免用强迫体位。

(3) Patient positioning: Normally select the sitting or recumbent position to make the treatment site optimally exposed and the patient in comfort.

（4）耐心解释，消除顾虑。对首次接受治疗的患者，要耐心解释药线点灸注意事项。壮医药线点灸疗法是一种既古老又新鲜的疗法，多数人对其并不了解，必须耐心把注意事项全面详细地向患者说明，以消除患者的顾虑，使患者能更好地配合治疗。

(4) Pre-operative instructions: Since the ZM medicated thread moxibustion, an

ancient therapy, is not well-known to people, give those who are treated with it for the first time the pre-operative instructions to eliminate their fears and worries. Thus, they can be cooperative.

（5）明确诊断，合理处方。抱着对患者高度负责的严肃态度，认真询问患者病史和自觉症状，一丝不苟地对其进行体格检查及相关的生化或影像检查，明确诊断，合理处方。

(5) Proper prescription: Meticulously inquire the patient's history of present illness and subjective symptoms and perform a physical assessment. If necessary, ask the patient to have biochemical or imaging tests. Make a diagnosis based on the collected information and examination results and accordingly write a proper prescription.

（二）操作流程
2　Operating procedure

壮医药线点灸疗法操作手法主要分整线、持线、点火、收线、施灸五步进行。

The operating procedure consists of 5 steps as follows.

第一步是整线。整线是把经药液浸泡后变松散的药线搓紧、拉直（图 8 ）。整线不仅可使点灸火力集中，还可减轻患者在点灸过程中的痛苦。

Step 1—medicated thread sorting: Tighten and straighten the loose strands of medicated thread after leaving it to soak in the decoction (Fig. 8). This enables the medicated thread to be more quickly ignited and the patient to feel less pain during moxibustion.

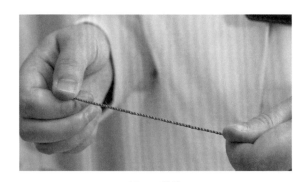

图 8　整线
Fig. 8　Medicated thread sorting

第二步是持线。持线是施术者用右手食指和拇指指尖相对，持药线一端，露出线头 1 ～ 2 cm（图 9）。露出的线头不能太短或太长，太短容易烧着施术者手指，太长不方便施灸操作。

Step 2—medicated thread holding: Hold the medicated thread with the right index finger and thumb fingertips (See Fig. 9). The distance between one end of the medicated thread and the fingers should be 1~2 cm long. If it is shorter than 1 cm, the practitioner's fingers are more likely to be burnt. If it is longer than 2 cm, it is not convenient to perform the moxibustion.

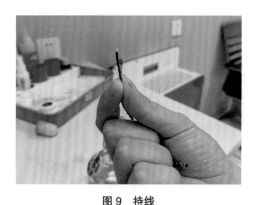

图 9　持线
Fig. 9　Medicated thread holding

第三步是点火。点火是将露出的线端在灯火上点燃，如有火苗必须抖灭，只需线头有圆珠状炭火星即可（图 10）。药线上的火苗必须轻柔地抖灭，不能用嘴巴吹灭。药线点燃后，一般会出现 4 种火候：一是明火，即有火焰；二是条火，即火焰熄灭后留下一条较长的药线炭火，不带火焰；三是珠火，即条火停留后，逐渐变小至线头呈圆珠状炭火星；四是径火，即珠火停留过久，逐渐变小，只有半边炭火星。以上 4 种火候中，只有珠火能够使用，其他 3 种火候不宜使用。若使用明火施灸，极易烧伤皮肤，出现水疱；使用条火施灸，很难对准穴位，且火力太强容易烫伤皮肤；使用径火施灸，药效及热量均不足，疗效欠佳。因此必须使用珠火点灸，以线端火星最旺时为点灸良机，以留在穴位上的药线炭灰呈白色为效果最好。

Step 3—ignition: Ignite the medicated thread from the end near the fingers (Fig. 10). When it is ignited, in the first place, there is an open fire on the end, which may propagate along the medicated thread and will become a smoldering fire. Then, when the smoldering fire goes out, the smoldered medicated thread will shrink to be a rounded spark which is gradually reduced to be a half-round spark. The open fire must be extinguished by gently shaking rather than by blowing. The open fire cannot be used for moxibustion because the skin can easily be burnt, causing blisters. Similarly, the strong smoldering fire makes the medicated thread hard to be aligned with the acupoints and tends to burn the skin so it is not suitable either. In contrast, the half-round spark is too weak to enable the medicine to work well. Only is the rounded spark suitable for moxibustion because it is strong enough to make the medicine have remarkable efficacy without burning the skin. Besides, the efficacy is optimal when the medicated thread ash on the acupoints is white.

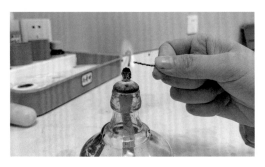

图 10　点火
Fig. 10　Ignition

第四步是收线。施术者持线手的小指先固定药线，中指和无名指再扣压药线，药线往回收的同时拇指适当往前伸，食指指尖与拇指指腹相对，露出线端 0.5 cm 即可，注意线头不能超出拇指的指尖。

Step 4—withdrawl: Wrap the medicated thread around the pinkie of one hand and hold it with the middle and ring fingers of the same hand. Then, buckle the medicated thread with the same hand's index finger tip and thumb pulp. Next, pull the medicated thread backwards while the thumb is moving towards until the distance between the thumb and one end of the medicated thread is 0.5 cm.

第五步是施灸。施术者将持线手固定在要施灸的穴位旁，将线头炭火星对准穴位。当线头炭火星变为圆珠状炭火星时，屈曲拇指指间关节将有圆珠状炭火星的线头直接扣压于穴位上，一按火灭即起为1壮，一般每穴点灸1～3壮（图11）。药线点灸操作的关键是顺应动作，拇指指腹稳重而又敏捷地将火星线头向下扣压，碰到穴位表面即行熄灭。

Step 5—moxibustion performance: Put the hand holding the medicated thread near the acupoint, with which the rounded spark is in line. Then, buckle the end on the acupoint by bending the thumb at its first interphalangeal joint. When the rounded spark goes out, a cone is counted (Fig. 11). Normally, 1~3 cones are applied to a point. It is worth emphasizing that the end should be pressed onto the point in the direction in which the wrist can be bent and with the thumb pulp quickly and steadily; and that the rounded spark should be immediately extinguished once the end touches the skin surface.

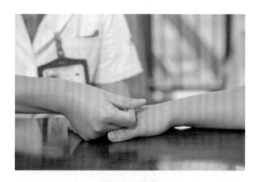

图 11　施灸
Fig. 11　Moxibustion performance

（三）注意事项

3　Cautions

壮医药线点灸疗法属于火灸、热灸，而且药线成分中含有麝香等药物，故在临床应用时必须注意以下事项。

The following rules should be obeyed since the moxibustion is applied by directly putting an ignited medicated thread which contains musk to the skin surface.

（1）必须严格掌握火候，切忌烧伤皮肤。药线点燃后，一般会出现4种火候，即明火、条火、珠火及径火。在以上4种火候中，只有珠火能够使用，其他3种火候不宜使用。

(1) Strictly control the heat to avoid skin burns. Among the four kinds of fire described above, keep in mind that only the rounded spark can be used for moxibustion.

（2）孕妇禁灸，尤其是其下半身穴位不能用药线点灸。

(2) Do not apply the moxibustion to a pregnant woman, especially to the acupoints on her lower body.

（3）眼球禁灸。

(3) Do not directly apply the moxibustion to the eyeballs.

（4）男性外生殖器龟头部和女性小阴唇部禁灸。

(4) Do not apply the moxibustion to the glans or labia minora.

（5）点灸眼区及面部靠近眼睛的穴位时，嘱患者闭目，以免不慎有火花飘入眼内引起烧伤。

(5) Ask the patient to close their eyes when the moxibustion is applied onto the acupoints on the eye area and the face near the eyes.

（6）患者情绪紧张或过度饥饿时慎灸。

(6) Use the therapy with caution when the patient is stressed or excessively hungry.

（7）点灸面部穴位时一律用轻手法。

(7) Gently put the medicated thread end onto the acupoints on the face.

（8）黑痣不宜用药线点灸，建议用药物或激光等做一次性彻底治疗。

(8) Do not use the therapy to treat moles, for which it is recommended to do a one-time thorough treatment with drugs or lasers.

（9）采用壮医药线点灸疗法后注意预防感染。穴位经药线点灸后，一般都有痒感，特别是同一穴位经连续数天点灸之后，局部会出现一个非常浅的灼伤痕迹，停止点灸1周左右即可自行消失。上述情况必须事先告诉患者，让其千万不要因为瘙痒或有灼伤而用手抓破施灸部位，以免引起感染。万一不小心抓破也不要紧，注意保持创口清洁，或用75%酒精消毒创口周围即可，不必惊慌。

(9) Tell patients the following possible expected situations prior to treatment: After moxibustion, itching will normally occur in the applied areas. If the moxibustion is applied on an acupoint for several consecutive days, a shallow burn mark will appear on the applied areas, but disappear in about a week after the treatment ends, so warn the patients not to scratch the itchy area or burnt area to

prevent infections. In case the skin in an applied area is broken by scratching, ask them to keep the wound clean or disinfect the area around the wound with 75% alcohol.

（10）注意嘱咐患者自觉配合治疗。治病是医生的责任，但同时也需要患者的密切配合。医生要认真做好咨询工作，有针对性地把一些疾病的基本常识告诉患者，调动患者的积极性，使其树立信心，自觉配合治疗。患者要遵照医嘱治疗，同时在饮食上有所忌口，如感冒患者必须连续点灸治疗 3 ～ 5 天；胃肠病患者在治疗期间要注意饮食，忌吃辛辣及肥甘厚味的食物；皮肤病患者必须忌食生葱、牛肉、马肉、母猪肉、海味、竹笋、韭菜、南瓜苗、公鸡肉、鲤鱼肉等发物。

(10) Ask patients to be cooperative because curing a disease is the responsibility of a practitioner, but also needs a patient's cooperation. Collect the information about patients' medical conditions as much as possible and tell them basic information about their disease to establish their confidence in curing it. This is conducive to making them be cooperative. Advise patients to accept the treatment as required. For example, those with cold should be treated for 3~5 days in a row. Also, advise them to avoid some foods if necessary. For example, those with gastrointestinal diseases should avoid spicy, greasy, sweet and salty foods during treatment. Those with skin diseases should avoid foods that make the medical conditions worse, including raw scallion, beef, horseflesh, sow pork, seafood, bamboo shoot, leek, pumkin seedling, rooster and carp.

四、常见病证治疗
Ⅳ　Treatment of common diseases

（一）嗘呗啷（带状疱疹）
1　Shingles ("Benbailang" in ZM)

1.疾病概述

1.1　General description

嗘呗啷是皮肤科和疼痛科一种常见疾病，是由水痘－带状疱疹病毒引起的，主要侵犯周围神经和皮肤，以周围神经疼痛和被侵犯神经所支配区域皮肤的红斑、丘疹、簇集性水疱疮为临床特征的一种皮肤感染性疾病。多见于一侧胸背或腰部皮肤出现集簇疱疹，常呈带状分布，伴剧烈辣痛，痛如火燎。因皮损状如蛇形，故又名蛇串疮；因多缠腰而发，故又名缠腰火丹、缠腰龙。多见于成年人，好发于春秋季节，相当于西医的带状疱疹。

Shingles ("Benbailang" in ZM) is a common disease treated by a dermatologist or pain management specialist. As a contagious skin disease, it is caused by varicella zoster virus which mainly attacks the peripheral nervous system and skin. Its clinical manifestations include pain in peripheral nerves and erythema, papules and vesicle clusters on the skin under which the nerves are invaded. Herpes clusters often appear in a band-like distribution on one side of the chest and back, or on the lower back and cause a sharp burning pain. Since skin lesions are often in a snake-like shape, it is also called herpes zoster, for which another name is zoster because it more often occurs in the lower back. It often develops in adults and occurs in spring and autumn.

2. 病因病机

1.2　Cause and mechanism of disease

湿热内蕴、复感火毒热邪为其病机特点。饮食失调，或脾失健运，湿浊内生，外发皮肤，聚于肌表；或情志不遂，郁久化热；或湿热内蕴，火热之毒，用于肌肤流窜三道两路，阻滞不通，故红斑、丘疹、疱疹、剧痛等症并见。

The mechanism of shingles is characterized by internal retention of dampness-heat accompanied by heat and pathogenic heat. An improper diet or dysfunction of the spleen in transportation leads to internal dampness turbidity which spreads to the skin and stagnates in the superficies. As a result, erythema, papules and herpes occur, accompanied by severe pain. These symptoms can also be caused by heat transformed from long-term excessive emotional activity. In addition, they appear when internal dampness-heat and heat travels along the superficies to block the three passages and two channels.

湿热邪毒入侵，日久阻滞龙路、火路，道路不通，气血运行不畅，耗散人体正气，人体正虚而祛邪无力，邪毒内蕴，毒壅于龙路、火路，阻滞不通，气血紊乱，可发为带状疱疹后遗神经痛。

Invasion of dampness-heat and/or pathogenic toxins block the dragon and fire channels, resulting in stagnation of qi and blood, which ultimately leads to excessive consumption of the healthy qi. The deficiency of the healthy qi disables the body to eliminate pathogenic factors. Thus, pathogenic toxins stagnate in the dragon and fire channels, leading to the blockage of these two channels. As a result, qi and blood are disharmonious, which will lead to postherpetic neuralgia.

3. 诊察要点

1.3　Essentials for diagnosis

（1）诊断依据。

(1) Diagnosis criteria.

① 主症。初起为发病部位辣痛，渐起为炎性红斑、红疹，并迅速转变为水疱，状似珍珠，疱液透亮，周围绕以红晕，数个水疱组成集簇状，排列成带状，伴有瘙痒、辣痛等症。经 1 周左右，疱液浑浊或部分溃破、糜烂、渗液，最后干燥结痂，待皮损脱落后，遗留瘢痕，部分患者有后遗神经痛达数月或数年之久。

① Main symptoms: At the onset, a burning pain occurs on the disease site. Gradually, inflammatory erythema and rashes appear and soon turn into pearl-like blisters that fill up with clear fluid. Clusters of blisters which look red around the borders often appear as a single stripe. They normally cause itching and a burning pain. After about 1 week, blister fluid become cloudy or some blisters break. Subsequently, the ruptured blisters are erosive with exudation and scab over. When the crusts fall off, scars remain in the place. Some patients experience postherpetic neuralgia, which can last for months or even years.

② 兼症。心烦易怒，夜不能寐，少气懒言，自汗，纳差，便溏，肢体困重，大便干，小便黄等。

② Concurrent symptoms: Vexation, irritability, sleeplessness, shortness of breath without desire to speak, spontaneous sweating, reduced appetite, loose stool, heavy sensation in the limbs, dry stool, yellow urine, etc.

③ 甲诊。指甲颜色青紫，按压甲尖后放开，久久未恢复原色，呈瘪螺甲、红紫甲或青斑甲。

③ Nail examination: The nails are bluish purple. When a fingernail stops being pressed, the color of the fingernail returns very slowly. Instead, the nail cap shrinks like a snail, reddish purple appears on the nail or there are blue spots on the nail.

④ 目诊。勒答上白睛脉络多而散乱，分布毫无规则。白睛脉络着色深为久病，脉络着色浅为新病；白睛脉络弯曲多、弯度大为病重、势急，脉络弯曲少、弯度小为病轻、势缓；白睛脉络粗大、红活、鲜红为实证，脉络细小、浅淡、色暗为虚证；白睛脉络边缘浸润混浊，边界不清，为挟有湿；白睛脉络散乱多为有风。

④ Eye examination: Many blood vessels on the white of the eyes are dilated, scattered and disordered. Dark-colored vessels mean long-term illness while light-colored ones mean short-term illness. Many large-radius bends on the vessels signify severe symptoms and abrupt onset while a few small-radius bends signify mild symptoms and slow onset. Bright red enlarged vessels indicate excess syndrome while dark-colored narrow ones at shallow depth indicate deficiency syndrome. The wet and turbid edges of the vessels show dampness which is one pathogenic factor of the disease while scattered and disordered vessels normally show wind which is one of the pathogenic factors.

（2）病证鉴别。

(2) Syndrome differentiation.

① 痤疮。痤疮是一种发于毛囊与皮脂腺的慢性炎症性皮肤病，因其临床表现包含粉刺，故又称粉刺。痤疮好发于青春期人群，临床主要表现为颜面、胸、背等处出现粟粒样丘疹如刺，或有囊肿、结节，有些融合成片，红肿或有脓头，可挤出白色或黄白色碎米样粉汁，伴有轻微瘙痒或疼痛。痤疮的病程往往较长，常此起彼伏，部分患者在青春期后可逐渐痊愈，但有些患者由于治疗不当或不注意卫生，可致其发为囊肿、结节或形成斑痕。

① Acne: Acne is a chronic inflammatory skin disease involving the hair follicles and sebaceous glands. This condition usually causes skin breakouts consisting of pimples. Its lesions also contain pimples. Therefore, acne is also known as pimple. It commonly occurs during puberty. The main clinical manifestations are millet-like papules, cysts or nodules on the face, chest and back. Some of them are in clusters. Normally, they are red and swollen, or filled with pus. They may cause slight itching or pain. When their walls break down, the white or yellowish sticky fluid will be discharged. Acne tends to run a long course because it waxes and wanes. Some patients can experience gradual recovery after puberty, but due to improper treatment or lack of hygiene, it will turn to nodular or cystic acne, or form scars.

诊断：颜面、胸、背等处出现粟粒样丘疹如刺，或有囊肿、结节，有些融合成片，红肿或者有脓头，伴有轻微瘙痒或疼痛，可挤出白色或黄白色碎米样粉汁；部分患处出现色素沉着。

Diagnosis criteria: Millet-like papules, cysts or nodules on the face, chest and back. Some of them are in clusters. They are red and swollen, or filled with pus. They may cause slight itching or pain. When their walls break down, the white or yellowish sticky fluid will be discharged. Pigmentation may appear in some affected areas.

② 湿疮。湿疮是指皮损呈多种形态，发无定位，易于湿烂渗液的一类瘙痒性渗出性皮肤病证，是一种常见的过敏性、炎症性皮肤病，好发于面部、肘窝、腘窝、四肢屈侧及躯干等处。湿疮由于患病部位不同而有不同的名称，如浸淫遍体、抓浸黄水、搔痒无度者，称为"浸淫疮"；以丘疹为主者，称为"血风疮"；发于阴囊部者，称为"肾囊风"；发于四肢弯曲部者，称为"四弯风"；发于婴幼儿颜面者，称为"奶癣"。男女老少均可发此病，无明显季节性，临床表现为皮损呈多样性，奇痒难忍，局部有渗出液，患处潮红或有红斑、丘疹、水疱、糜烂、痂皮。疤痕处易反复发作。

② Eczema: Eczema is a common allergic inflammatory skin disease characterized by variable forms of skin lesion, exudation and intense pruritus. It can occur on any part of the body, but is most common on the face, cubital fossa, popliteal fossa, flexural surfaces of the extremities and torso. Eczema has different names on different areas. For example, exudative eczema is characterized by erythema on any part of the body, associated with serous exudate and extreme itching; general papular eczema is characterized by papules; scrotal eczema refers to eczema of the scrotum; cubito-popliteal eczema means eczema occurs in the cubital and popliteal fossae; and milk dematomycosis is another name for infantile eczema normally occurring in a baby's face. Eczema can appear at any age and in any season. It can lead to many kinds of skin damage, including intense pruritus, serous exudate, redness, erythema, papules, blisters, erosion and scarring which tends to recur.

诊断：急性湿疮，表现为皮肤红斑、丘疹、水疱兼夹，集簇成片状，因搔抓常引起糜烂、渗出、结痂等，边缘不清，常成对称分布。慢性湿疮，表现为皮肤肥厚粗糙，皮沟明显，可呈苔藓样变，颜色褐红色或褐色，表面常附有糠皮状鳞屑，伴有抓痕、结痂及色素沉着等。一般全身症状及体征不明显，部分患者可有烦躁不安、失眠、情绪紧张等表现。

Diagnosis criteria: Acute eczema is characterized by clusters of erythema, papules and blisters which are symmetrically distributed and cause itching, erosion due to scratching, watery discharge and the development of crusts; chronic eczema is marked by thickened skin with obvious grooves, lichenification, maroon or brown skin, bran-like scales, scratch marks, scar formation and pigmentation; and normally, the signs and symptoms are not noticeable. Some patients experience irritability, insomnia and stress.

4. 辨证论治

1.4　Syndrome differentiation and treatment

（1）治疗原则。祛湿通络，清热解毒，调气止痛，通龙路火路。

(1) Treatment principles. Dispel dampness to unblock the collaterals, clear away heat, resolve toxins, adjust qi to relieve pain and unblock the dragon and fire channels.

（2）证治分类。

(2) Classification of syndrome identification and treatment.

① 选穴原则。采用壮医"痒疾抓长子""寒手热背肿在梅"的配穴原则。"痒疾抓长子"，即选取首先出现的疱疹或最大的疱疹进行点灸；"寒手"，即凡出现畏寒发冷症状，取手部穴位为主；"热背"，即凡出现发热症状，取背部穴位为主；"肿在梅"，即凡出现肿块或皮损，则沿肿块或皮损的边缘和中心点取一组穴位组成梅花形。在治疗过程中，随着肿块和皮损的缩小，梅花形穴的外周取穴也跟着移动。

① Principles of acupoints selection: The medicated thread moxibustion is applied to acupoints according to different medical conditions. Specifically, for the treatment of skin itching due to rash-type diseases, points on the area, where rashes first appeared or the largest rash is, are selected as the primary ones; points on the hands are selected to treat those with fear of cold and chills; points on the back are selected for those with a fever; to treat bumps or skin lesions, normally, four specific points along the edge of the bump or lesion and one point in its center are used. During treatment, different points along the edge will be selected with the reduction of bumps and skin lesions.

② 主穴。阿是穴、长子穴、局部梅花穴、内关、曲池、足三里、血海等。

② Primary acupoints: Ashi points, points on the area where rashes first appeared or the largest rash is, a point in the affected area with other points on its corner, which looks like a plum flower, Neiguan (PC 6), Quchi (LI 11), Zusanli (ST 36), Xuehai (SP 10).

③ 辨证分型选穴。

③ Acupoints selection after syndrome differentiation.

阳证（带状疱疹）。发病前常伴有一些全身症状，如倦怠、少食、发热、头痛等，其潜伏期为 7 ～ 12 天。初起为发病部位辣痛，渐起为出现炎性红斑、红疹，并迅速转变为水疱，状似珍珠，疱液透亮，周围绕以红晕，数个水疱组成集簇状，排列成带状，伴有瘙痒、辣痛等症。经 1 周左右，疱液浑浊或部分溃破、糜烂、渗液，最后干燥结痂，待皮损脱落后，遗留瘢痕。

Yang syndrome (shingles): There are some symptoms prior to the onset of the disease, including lassitude, reduced appetite, fever and headache. The incubation period of the disease usually is between seven and twelve days. Initially, a burning pain occurs on the disease site. Gradually, inflammatory erythema and rashes appear and soon turn into pearl-like blisters filled with clear fluid. Clusters of blisters that look red around the borders often appear as a single stripe. They normally cause itching and a burning pain. After about 1 week, blister fluid become cloudy or some blisters break. Subsequently, the ruptured blisters are erosive with exudation and scab over. When the crusts fall off, scars remain in the place.

此为湿热型。主症：皮肤潮红，出现丘疹、丘疱疹、水疱、糜烂、渗液；自觉灼热、瘙痒，可伴有心烦，口渴，舌红，苔黄，脉滑数。

Dampness-heat type. Main symptoms: Redness, papules, papulovesicles, blisters, erosion, exudate, which cause a burning sensation and pruritus, accompanied by vexation and thirst, red tongue with yellow coating and slippery pulse.

治疗原则：清热毒，利湿毒，调气止痛。

Treatment principles: Clear away heat, remove dampness and adjust qi to relieve pain.

取穴：阿是穴、长子穴、局部梅花穴、内关、曲池等。

Acupoints selection: Ashi points, points on the area where rashes first appeared or the largest rash is, a point in the affected area with other points on its corner, which looks like a plum flower, Neiguan (PC 6) and Quchi (LI 11).

阴证（带状疱疹后遗神经痛）。好发于中老年人、免疫力低下者及有带状疱疹发病史者。带状疱疹的皮疹消退后，局部皮肤略有疼痛不适，且持续一个月以上。临床表现为局部阵发性或持续性的灼痛、刺痛、跳痛、刀割痛，严重者影响休息睡眠及精神状态等，其发生率随年龄增长而提高。

Yin syndrome (postherpetic neuralgia): Postherpetic neuralgia often occurs in middle-aged and elderly people, immunocompromised people, and people with a medical history of shingles. When shingles rashes resolve, discomfort in the skin of some disease sites may be manifested as a burning pain, a stabbing pain, a throbbing pain and a cutting pain, which are persistent or intermittent. The pain normally lasts for at least one month. If the pain is severe, sleep quality and the mental state will be affected. The prevalence of postherpetic neuralgia increases with aging.

若为脾虚湿困型，则主症：皮损色淡或褐色，出现红斑、丘疹、丘疱疹、少量渗液或皮肤肥厚、粗糙；自觉瘙痒，可伴有食少，腹胀便溏，舌淡胖，苔腻，脉濡或滑。

Spleen deficiency with dampness. Main symptoms: Light-colored or brown skin lesions, erythema, papule and/or papulovesicles, which have a small amount of watery discharge or make the skin thickened, pruritus that may be accompanied by reduced appetite, abdomen distension and loose stool, pale and plump tongue with greasy coating and soggy or slippery pulse.

治疗原则：健脾胃，除湿毒，调气止痛。

Treatment principles: Invigorate the spleen and stomach, remove dampness and adjust qi to relieve pain.

取穴：局部梅花穴、足三里、手三里、合谷、曲池等。

Acupoints selection: A point in the affected area with other points on its corner, which looks like a plum flower, Zusanli (ST 36), Shousanli (LI 10), Hegu (LI 4) and Quchi (LI 11).

若为阴虚血燥型，则主症：皮损肥厚粗糙，苔藓样变，具鳞屑，色素沉着；自觉阵发性瘙痒，夜间加重，可伴心烦失眠，舌淡红，脉弦细。

Pattern of yin deficiency with blood dryness. Main symptoms: Thickened skin lesions, scales, lichenification, pigmentation, intermittent pruritus which becomes worse at night, often accompanied by vexation, insomnia, reddish tongue and wiry, thready pulse.

治疗原则：养血祛风，化湿通络，调气止痛。

Treatment principles: Nourish blood, dispel wind, resolve dampness to unblock the collaterals and adjust qi to relieve pain.

取穴：局部梅花穴、血海、三阴交、足三里、太溪等。

Acupoints selection: A point in the affected area with other points on its corner, which looks like a plum flower, Xuehai (SP 10), Sanyinjiao (SP 6), Zusanli (ST 36) and Taixi (KI 3).

5. 预防调护

1.5　Prevention and care

忌用热水烫洗施灸部位和用肥皂等刺激物洗澡；尽量避免用力抓挠施灸部位；饮食宜清淡有节，忌食辛辣食物及鸡肉、羊肉、牛肉、鱼肉、海鲜等发物，少吃油腻甜食等；戒烟酒，起居有常，保持睡眠充足。

Do not take a shower with hot water or stimulants such as soap. Do not scratch the skin hard. Have a bland diet regularly. Avoid foods that make the medical conditions worse, including chicken, lamb, beef, fish or seafood. Cut down on greasy and sweet foods. Quit smoking and alcohol consumption. Live a regular life to ensure adequate sleep.

6. 医案选读

1.6　Selected case readings

【病案一】

［Case 1］

李某，男，47 岁，2019 年 7 月 2 日初诊。

Patient: Li, a 47-year-old man; his first visit was on July 2, 2019.

主诉：左上肢内侧、左肩胛及左掌心出现疱疹 6 天，伴有瘙痒、灼痛感。

Chief complaint:"Blisters appeared on the inside of my left upper limb, left scapula and palm 6 days ago. They caused pruritus and a burning sensation."

现病史：患者 2019 年 6 月底出现不明诱因的左上肢内侧、左肩胛及左掌心疼痛不适，6 天后出现疱疹，瘙痒难忍，灼痛难耐，疱疹集簇成片，并有少许渗液，左掌心尤为严重。伴大便溏烂、睡眠不安。舌质红，舌苔厚白而腻，脉弦。

History of present illness: Pain occurred in the inside of the patient's left upper limb, left scapula and palm at the end of June 2019. Six days later, clusters of blister appeared, accompanied by pruritus, a burning sensation and a small amount of exudation. These symptoms were more obvious in the left palm. He reported loose stools and poor sleep quality.His tongue is red with thick, pale and greasy coating. His pulse is wiry.

壮医诊断：喯呗啷（阳证）。中医诊断：蛇串疮。西医诊断：带状疱疹。

Diagnosis in ZM:"Benbailang" characterized by yang syndrome.

Diagnosis in TCM: Herpes zoster.

Diagnosis in WM: Shingles.

治疗原则：清热利湿，行气止痛。

Treatment principles: Clear away heat, induce dampness and move qi to relieve pain.

治疗：壮医药线点灸疗法。取局部莲花穴、长子穴、内关、血海、胸龙脊、肩井等穴位。每穴点灸 3 壮，每天点灸 1 次。连续治疗 10 天后，疱疹结痂，疼痛消失。

Therapeutic methods: The ZM medicated thread moxibustion.

Acupoints selection: Points in the affected area, which look like a lotus, points on the area where rashes first appeared or the largest rash is, Neiguan (PC 6), Xuehai (SP 10), points on the thoracic spine and Jianjing (GB 21). 1~3 cones are applied to a point, one time per day. After ten consecutive days of treatment, the patient's herpes crusted over and pain disappeared.

【病案二】

［Case 2］

刘某，男，73 岁，2020 年 9 月 13 日初诊。

Patient: Liu, a 73-year-old man; his first visit was on September 13, 2020.

主诉：右侧额面三叉神经分布区域针刺样痛 8 年。

Chief complaint:"I have experienced a stabbing pain in the distribution of my right frontal trigeminal nerve for 8 years."

现病史：患者于 2012 年无明显诱因下右侧颌部出现带状疱疹，在当地医院行抗病毒等治疗后，疱疹消失，但遗留右侧三叉神经痛，呈针刺样痛，痛时难耐。当年行神经阻断切除治疗，疗效不佳，每次痛时均靠服用卡马西平止痛，连服 8 年。刻下症见右侧额面三叉神经分布区域针刺样痛，不能触碰，夜间疼痛加剧，风吹、洗脸时疼痛难耐，痛时涕泪俱下，每日服卡马西平 4 片止痛，不能戒断，并出现手脚皮肤增厚、粗糙现象。肝功能检查提示轻度肝损害。头颅磁共振检查提示轻度脑萎缩。舌质暗红，舌苔黄腻，脉滑数。

History of present illness: Shingles occurred on the right side of the patient's jaw in 2012 without any apparent reasons. After being treated with antivirus drugs at a local hospital, herpes disappeared, but trigeminal neuralgia in his right face remained. He described it as an intolerable stabbing pain. In 2012, he was treated with therapeutic nerve blocks but the pain was not much relieved, so he had to take carbamazepine to relieve pain when it occurred every time in the past 8 years. When he sought medical care at our hospital, his main symptom was a stabbing pain in the distribution of his right frontal trigeminal nerve which could not be touched. He reported the pain became worse at night and intolerable when the wind blew on his face or he washed his face. The pain made him suffer from a snotty nose and runny eyes. He had to take 4 tablets of carbamazepine daily to maintain pain relief. His hand and foot skins have thickened and rough. His tongue is dark red with yellow, greasy coating. His pulse is slippery and rapid. The results of his liver function tests indicate mild liver damage. Mild brain atrophy is seen on his brain MRI.

壮医诊断：嘈呗嘟（阴证）。中医诊断：蛇串疮。西医诊断：带状疱疹后遗神经痛。

Diagnosis in ZM:"Benbailang" characterized by yin syndrome.

Diagnosis in TCM: Herpes zoster.

Diagnosis in WM: Postherpetic neuralgia.

治疗原则：调和气血，祛风止痛。

Treatment principles: Harmonize qi and blood, dispel wind and relieve pain.

治疗：壮医药线点灸疗法。取局部葵花穴、百会、安眠三穴（神门、安眠、三阴交，双侧）、颊车（双侧）、大椎、肩井、合谷、内关等穴位。每穴点灸3壮（图 12）。每周点灸 2～3 次，10 次为 1 个疗程。经药线点灸治疗 3 次后，疼痛减轻，洗脸时再无涕泪俱下的情况；继续治疗 1 个月，经药线点灸治疗 12 次后，疼痛继续减轻，由原来每天服用卡马西平 4 片减少为每天只服用 2 片；继续治疗 3 个月，经药线点灸治疗 30 次后，停服卡马西平，疼痛消失；随访半年，除劳累时局部仍有一些不适外，疗效持久。

Therapeutic methods: The medicated thread moxibustion.

Acupoints selection: Points in the affected area, which look like a sunflower, Baihui (GV 20), Shenmen (HT 7), Anmian (EX-HN 22) and Sanyinjiao (SP 6) on extremities, Jiache (ST 6) on both cheeks, Dazhui (GV 14), Jianjing (GB 21), Hegu (LI 4) and Neiguan (PC 6).

Treatment frequency: 3 cones are applied to each point (Fig. 12), 2~3 times of treatment per week with 10 times of treatment is a treatment course.

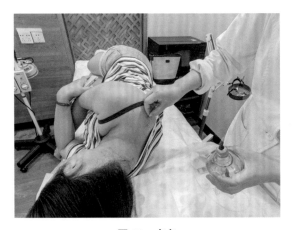

图 12　点灸

Fig. 12　The medicated thread moxibustion

After 3 times of treatment, the pain was relieved. The patient did not suffer from a snotty nose and runny eyes when he washed his face. After twelve times of treatment within a month, the pain was further relieved so he only needed to take two tablets of carbamazepine daily. After thirty times of treatment within three months, the pain disappeared so he stopped taking the drug. In a half year follow-up, he reported there was merely local discomfort in some areas when he was tired and the efficacy remained high.

（二）麦蛮 / 笨隆（风疹）

2　Rubella ("Maiman/Benlong" in ZM)

1. 疾病概述

2.1　General description

麦蛮 / 笨隆属壮医风毒病。中医称之为"瘾疹""风疹块"，相当于现代医学的风疹。麦蛮 / 笨隆是皮肤出现时隐时现的风团的一类瘙痒性、过敏性皮肤病，临床特点是皮肤上出现风团，色红或白，形状不规则，边界清楚，稍高于皮肤，瘙痒难忍，发无定处，骤起骤退，退后不留痕迹，可伴头晕、发热、恶心、呕吐、纳食减少等。好发于冬春季，尤以儿童发病为多见。

From the perspective of ZM, rubella, also known as "Maiman/Benlong" in ZM, hives in TCM and urticaria in WM, is a disease caused by wind. It is an allergic disorder of the skin, marked by red or pale wheals and intermittent pruritus. The wheals are intensely itchy, raised patches in an irregular shape but with clearly defined edges. They can occur on any part of the body, suddenly wax and wane but without a trace behind. They can cause dizziness, fever, nausea, vomiting and reduced appetite. Rubella occurs more often in spring and winter, with a higher frequency in children.

2. 病因病机

2.2　Cause and mechanism of disease

壮医认为，本病是风毒入侵人体肌肤，游走不定或结于局部，阻滞龙路火路，气机不畅而致。

From the perspective of ZM, rubella is caused by stagnation of qi movement because the dragon and fire channels are blocked by wind which runs through the body or stagnates at a local area after attacking the skin.

3. 诊察要点

2.3 Essentials for diagnosis

（1）诊断依据。

(1) Diagnosis criteria.

① 参照《中国壮医学》中风毒病之风疹的诊断标准拟定。

① The diagnosis criteria for rubella caused by wind are outlined according to *China's Zhuang Medicine.*

主症：皮肤出现红色斑块，形状不规则，边界清楚，稍高于皮肤，瘙痒难忍，此起彼伏。

Main symptoms: Raised red skin bumps, in an irregular shape but with clearly defined edges, characteristic of pruritus, on and off.

兼症：头晕，发热，恶心，呕吐，纳食减少，腹痛，腹泻，呼吸困难等。

Concurrent symptoms: Dizziness, fever, nausea, vomiting, reduced appetite, abdominal pain, diarrhea and shortness of breath.

甲诊：指甲颜色青紫，按压甲尖后放开，久久未恢复原色，呈瘪螺甲、红紫甲或青斑甲。

Nail examination: The fingernails are bluish purple. When a fingernail stops being pressed, the color of the fingernail return very slowly. Instead, the nail cap shrinks like a snail, reddish purple appears on the nail or there are blue spots on the nail.

目诊：勒答上白睛脉络多而散乱，分布无规则。

Eye examination: Many blood vessels on the white of the eyes are dilated, scattered and disordered.

② 参照中华人民共和国中医药行业标准《中医皮肤科病证诊断疗效标准》（ZY/T001. 8—1994）。

② According to *The Standards of Diagnosis and Assessment of Treatment Efficacy of Dermatological Conditions in Traditional Chinese Medicine (ZY/T001.8—1994)*, the diagnosis criteria include.

发病突然，皮损为大小不等、形状不一的水肿性斑块，边界清楚。

Rubella starts with a sudden onset of edematous plaques of varying sizes and shapes but with clearly defined edges.

皮疹时起时落，剧烈瘙痒，发无定处，消退后不留痕迹。

Wheals are on and off, characteristic of intense pruritus. They occur on any part of the body and disappear without a trace.

发作，常迁延不愈。

Rubella are recurrent and often irresponsible to treatment.

③参照《临床诊疗指南：皮肤病与性病分册》（中华医学会编著，人民卫生出版社，2006 年）和《中国临床皮肤病学》（赵辨主编，江苏凤凰科学技术出版社，2010 年）。

③ According to *The Guidelines for the Clinical Diagnosis and Treatment of Skin and Venereal Diseases* compiled by the Chinese Medical Association and published by the People's Medical Publishing House in 2006 and *China Clinical Dermatology* edited by Zhao Bian and published by the Phoenix Science Press in 2010, the diagnosis criteria include.

皮疹为大小不等的风团，色鲜红，也可为苍白色，孤立散在或融合成片，数小时内风团减轻，变为红斑而逐渐消失。但不断有新的风团出现。

Red or pale wheals in irregular shapes are scattered or in clusters. They turn to be red spots and disappear but reappear within hours.

全身症状一般较轻，风团时多时少，反复发生，病程在 6 周以上。

The symptoms are usually mild. Wheals can vary in quantities and recur. They may persist for more than 6 weeks.

（2）病证鉴别。

(2) Syndrome differentiation.

①丘疹性荨麻疹。本病为散在性、性质稍坚硬、顶端有小疱的丘疹，周围有纺锤形红晕，自觉瘙痒。本病瘙痒剧烈，多数被认为与昆虫叮咬有关。儿童多见。

① Papular urticaria. Papular urticaria is defined by eruption of slightly hard itchy papules. A pustule is at the top of each papule with spindle-shaped redness along its edge. The disease is characterized by intense pruritus and an allergic skin reaction to insect bites or stings. It is more often seen in children.

② 阑尾炎。伴有腹痛的风疹需要与外科急腹症如阑尾炎等相区别。后者右下腹疼痛较显著，有压痛，白细胞总数和中性粒细胞比例明显增加。

② Appendicitis. Urticaria with abdominal pain needs to be differentiated from acute abdomen such as appendicitis. Appendicitis causes obvious pain, which is aggravated by pressure. The pain is more obvious in the lower right abdomen. White blood cell counts and neutrophil level are abnormally elevated.

4. 辨证论治

2.4　Syndrome differentiation and treatment

（1）治疗原则。疏通两路气机，驱风排毒止痒。

(1) Treatment principles. Move qi in the two channels, dispel wind and remove toxins to relieve itching.

（2）证治分类。

(2) Classification of syndrome identification and treatment.

① 选穴原则。采用壮医"痒疾抓长子""寒手热背肿在梅"的配穴原则。"痒疾抓长子"，即选取首先出现的风疹或最大的风疹进行点灸；"寒手"，即凡出现畏寒发冷症状，以取手部穴位为主；"热背"，即凡出现发热症状，以取背部穴位为主；"肿在梅"，即凡出现肿块或皮损，则沿肿块或皮损的边缘和中心点取一组穴位组成梅花形。在治疗过程中，随着肿块和皮损的缩小，梅花形穴的外周取穴也跟着移动。

① Principles of acupoints selection: The medicated thread moxibustion is applied to acupoints according to different medical conditions. Specifically, for the treatment of skin itching due to rash-type diseases, points on the area, where rashes first appeared or the largest rash is, are selected as the primary ones; points on the hands are selected to treat those with fear of cold and chills; points on the back are selected for those with a fever; to treat bumps or skin lesions, normally, four specific points along the edge of the bump or lesion and one point in its center are used. During treatment, different points along the edge are selected with the reduction of bumps and skin lesions.

② 主穴。阿是穴、长子穴、三阴交、曲池、足三里、手三里、血海、局部梅花穴。

② Primary acupoints: Ashi points, points on the area where rashes first appeared or the largest rash is, Sanyinjiao (SP 6), Quchi (LI 11), Zusanli (ST 36), Shousanli (LI 10), Xuehai (SP 10) and a point in the affected area with other points on its corner, which looks like a plum flower.

③ 辨证分型选穴。

③ Acupoints selection after syndrome differentiation.

阴证。若为风寒外袭，则主症：风团色白，遇寒加重，得暖则减；恶寒，口不渴；舌淡红，苔薄白，脉浮紧。

Yin syndrome. External wind-cold attack. Symptoms: Pale wheals which increase due to cold and decrease due to heat, aversion to cold, absence of thirst, light red tongue with white, thin coating, and floating, tight pulse.

取穴：长子穴、局部梅花穴、曲池、合谷、血海、膈俞。

Acupoints selection: Points on the area where rashes first appeared or the largest rash is, a point in the affected area with other points on its corner, which looks like a plum flower, Quchi (LI 11), Hegu (LI 4), Xuehai (SP 10) and Geshu (BL 17).

若为血虚风燥，则主症：反复发作，迁延日久，午后或夜间加剧；伴心烦易怒，口干，手足心热，舌红少津，脉沉细。

Blood deficiency and wind-dryness. Symptoms: Recurrent, refractory wheals which increase in the afternoon or at night, accompanied by vexation, irritability and thirst, and feverish sensation in the palms and soles, red tongue with little saliva and deep, thready pulse.

取穴：长子穴、局部梅花穴、大肠俞、肺俞、曲池、足三里。

Acupoints selection: Points on the area where rashes first appeared or the largest rash is, a point in the affected area with other points on its corner, which looks like a plum flower, Dachangshu (BL 25), Feishu (BL 13), Quchi (LI 11) and Zusanli (ST 36).

阳证。胃肠积热。主症：风团片大色红，瘙痒剧烈；发疹的同时伴脘腹疼痛，恶心呕吐，神疲纳呆，大便秘结或泄泻；舌质红，苔黄腻，脉弦滑数。

Yang syndrome. Gastrointestinal heat retention. Symptoms: Intensely pruritic, red wheals in large clusters, accompanied by abdominal pain, nausea, vomiting, fatigue and constipation or diarrhea, red tongue with yellow and greasy coating, wiry, slippery and rapid pulse.

取穴：长子穴、局部梅花穴、曲池、足三里、脾俞、三阴交。

Acupoints selection: Points on the area where rashes first appeared or the largest rash is, a point in the affected area with other points on its corner, which looks like a plum flower, Quchi (LI 11), Zusanli (ST 36), Pishu (BL 20) and Sanyinjiao (SP 6).

④ 穴位加减。若以上半身瘙痒为主，则加风池、大椎、合谷。若以下半身瘙痒为主，则加委中、阴陵泉。若反复发作，久病难愈，则加关元、气海、百会、脾俞。

④ Modification: For intense pruritus mainly occurring in the upper body, add Fengchi (GB 20), Dazhui (GV 14) and Hegu (LI 4). For intense pruritus mainly occurring in the lower body, add Weizhong (BL 40) and Yinlingquan (SP 9). For recurrence and irresponsibility to treatment, add Guanyuan (CV 4), Qihai (CV 6), Baihui (GV 20) and Pishu (BL 20).

（3）疗程。每日 1～2 次，5 次为 1 个疗程。

2.4.3　Treatment course: 1~2 times daily, 5 times is a treatment course.

5. 预防调护

2.5　Prevention and care

（1）患者应避免进食鱼虾类食物和含有人工色素、防腐剂、酵母菌等的罐头、腌腊食品、饮料等。

(1) Avoid fish, shrimps, canned foods containing artificial pigments, preservatives and yeasts, pickled food and soft drinks.

（2）患者应保持在室内外都处于清洁卫生的环境中，避免吸入花粉、粉尘等。家中不养猫、狗之类的宠物。

(2) Keep the house clean to avoid inhaling pollen and dust. Do not keep hairy animals such as dogs and cats.

（3）平时生活规律，适当运动，增强体质，可减少发病机会。

(3) Live a regular life and work out regularly to strengthen the body and reduce

the possibility of be attacked by rubella.

（4）喝酒、受热、情绪激动、用力等都会加重皮肤血管扩张，激发或加重症状，应当尽量避免。

(4) Avoid alcohol consumption, heat, excess emotional activity and physical exertion, which dilate blood vessels in the skin, thereby triggering or worsening the symptoms.

（5）患冷性风疹者不要去海水浴场，也不能洗冷水浴，冬季要注意保暖。

(5) For those with rubella caused by exposure to cold, avoid sea bathing and cold showers, and keep themselves warm in winter.

（6）积极治疗有可能诱发风疹的疾病，如肠道蛔虫病、蛲虫病、龋齿、扁桃体炎、中耳炎、鼻窦炎、癣病等。

(6) Treat diseases that may cause rubella in time, including intestinal ascariasis, enterobiasis, dental caries, tonsillitis, otitis media, sinusitis and ringworm.

（7）保持健康心态，提高身体免疫力。

(7) Keep a healthy mind to boost the body's natural defenses.

6. 医案选读

2.6　Selected case readings

【病案一】

［Case 1］

陈某，男，40 岁，2020 年 8 月 13 日就诊。

Patient: Chen, a 40-year-old man, his first visit was on August 13, 2020.

现病史：患者于昨天饮酒后，全身突发大片风团，瘙痒剧烈，以头面、躯干为著，色红或赤，遇热则痒甚，皮疹退而复发，伴脘腹疼痛、恶心、大便稀烂秽臭。患者以往多次出现类似病证，每予抗组胺类药物口服治疗后皮疹消退而愈。本次再发，经口服氯雷他定、西替利嗪仍有皮疹。发病以来无胸闷、气喘。

History of present illness: After drinking yesterday, red or crimson wheals in large clusters occurred all over the patient's body, especially on his head, face and torso. They caused pruritus, which was worsened by heat. Being on and off, they caused abdominal pain and nausea, loose and smelly stools. He reported that he had had similar diseases previously, which had been cured with oral administration of antihistamine. However, the wheals did not disappear after he took loratadine and cetirizole this time. He had no thoracic oppression or shortness of breath.

查体：一般情况可。头面、前胸、两上肢见红色或赤色风团，或散在，或联合成片，大小不一，压之褪色。舌质红，苔黄腻，脉滑数。

Physical examination: The visual body check shows the patient's medical conditions are not bad. Red or crimson wheals are scattered or in clusters on his head, face, the anterior side of his chest and two upper extremities. They are in an irregular shape and fades under pressure. His tongue is red with yellow, greasy coating. His pulse is slippery and rapid.

甲诊：指甲颜色红紫，按压甲尖后放开，久久未恢复原色。

Nail examination: The patient's fingernails are reddish purple. When a fingernail stops being pressed, the color will return very slowly.

目诊：勒答上白睛脉络多而散乱，分布无规则。

Eye examination: Many blood vessels on the white of the eyes are dilated, scattered and disordered.

诊断：风疹（阳证－胃肠积热）。

Diagnosis: Rubella, characterized by gastrointestinal heat retention, a type of yang syndrome.

治疗：壮医药线点灸疗法。

Treatment method: The ZM medicated thread moxibustion.

取穴：局部梅花穴、长子穴、大椎、合谷、曲池、足三里、脾俞、三阴交。每日 2 次。治疗 3 天后，皮疹消退。继续取穴曲池、足三里、脾俞、三阴交。每日 1 次，巩固疗效治疗 3 次。

Acupoints selection: A point in the affected area with other points on its corner, which looks like a plum flower, points on the area where rashes first appeared or the largest rash is, Dazhui (GV 14), Hegu (LI 4), Quchi (LI 11), Zusanli (ST 36), Pishu (BL 20) and Sanyinjiao (SP 6). The therapy was applied twice daily. After three days, wheals disappeared. It continued to be applied on Quchi (LI 11), Zusanli (ST 36), Pishu (BL 20) and Sanyinjiao (SP 6) one time daily, three times in total, to consolidate the efficacy.

【病案二】

［Case 2］

张某，女，50 岁，2021 年 2 月 5 日就诊。

Patient: Zhang, a 50-year-old woman, her first visit was on February 5, 2021.

现病史：患者于 5 天前受凉后出现鼻塞流清涕、咽痒、打喷嚏等症状，自服感冒药后症状减轻。于前天全身散见风团，色淡红或白，皮疹瘙痒，遇风则加重，得暖则减轻。伴有恶风寒、头疼，口不渴。

History of present illness: Five days ago, the patient had a cold which caused a stuffy and runny nose, itchy throat and sneezing. These symptoms were eased after she took cold medicines. The day before yesterday, light red or pale wheals appeared all over her body. They cause pruritus which was worsened by wind but relieved by heat. She reported aversion to cold and wind, headache, and absence of thirst.

查体：一般情况可。头面、躯干散见淡红色或白色风团，呈斑片状，大小不一、边界清楚。舌淡，苔薄白，脉浮紧。

Physical examination: The visual body check shows the patient's medical conditions are not bad. Patches of light red or pale wheals are scattered on her head, face and torso. These patches vary in size but with clearly defined edges. Her tongue is pale with white, thin coating. Her pulse is floating and tight.

甲诊：指甲颜色青紫，按压甲尖后放开，久久未恢复原色。

Nail examination: The fingernails are bluish purple. When a fingernail stops being pressed, the color of the fingernail will return very slowly.

目诊：勒答上白睛脉络多而散乱，分布无规则。

Eye examination: Many blood vessels on the white of the eyes are dilated, scattered and disordered.

诊断：风疹（阴证－风寒外袭）。

Diagnosis: Rubella, characterized by external wind-cold attack, a type of yin syndrome.

治疗：壮医药线点灸疗法。

Treatment method: The ZM medicated thread moxibustion.

取穴：局部梅花穴、长子穴、曲池、合谷、血海、膈俞。每日 2 次。

Acupoints selection: A point in the affected area with other points on its corner, which looks like a plum flower, points on the area where rashes first appeared or the largest rash is, Quchi (LI 11), Hegu (LI 4), Xuehai (SP 10) and Geshu (BL 17). The therapy was applied twice daily.

治疗 2 天后，皮疹减少，复发时间延长，伴有恶风、乏力（图 13）。取穴：局部梅花穴、大椎、风池、曲池、合谷、血海、膈俞。每日 2 次。治疗 3 天后，皮疹完全消退。继续取穴曲池、合谷、血海、膈俞。每日 1 次，巩固疗效治疗 3 次。

After two days, wheals decreased and the recurrence interval became longer (Fig. 13). She reported aversion to cold and lassitude. Therefore, the therapy was applied twice daily. The selected acupoints included a point in the affected area with other points on its corner, which looks like a plum flower, Dazhui (GV 14), Fengchi (GB 20), Quchi (LI 11), Hegu (LI 4), Xuehai (SP 10) and Geshu (BL 17). After three days, wheals disappeared. In order to consolidate the efficacy, the therapy continued to be applied once daily in three consecutive days, using Quchi (LI 11), Hegu (LI 4), Xuehai (SP 10) and Geshu (BL 17).

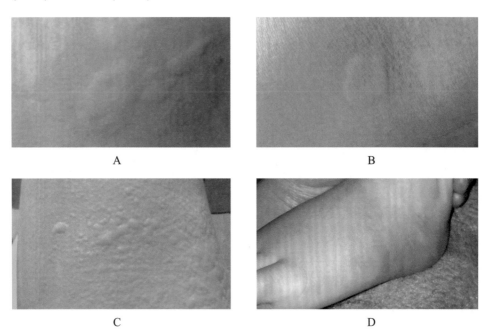

A

B

C

D

图 13　皮疹

Fig. 13　wheals

（三）巧尹（头痛）

3　Headache ("Qiaoyin" in ZM)

1. 疾病概述

3.1　General description

巧尹是指外感或内伤致巧坞不利而引起的以自觉头部疼痛为主要症状的一种疾病。其可单独出现，亦可见于多种其他疾病，可表现为整个头部疼痛或头的后部、偏侧部疼痛。

"Qiaoyin" is a common pain in the head affected by external contraction or endogenous damage. It can occur alone or with other symptoms across the head or on the back and two sides of the head.

巧尹相当于中医的头痛；西医的颈椎病、高血压、偏头痛、血管神经性头痛、紧张性头痛及一些五官科疾病等，也可参考本病进行诊治。

"Qiaoyin" is also known as headache in TCM. Treatment for diseases in WM, including cervical spondylosis, hypertension, migraine, angioneurotic headache, tension headache and some ENT diseases, can refer to the ZM treatment methods applied to "Qiaoyin".

2. 病因病机

3.2　Cause and mechanism of disease

巧尹的发病与外感风、寒、湿或内伤肝、脾、肾三脏有关。常见原因为风邪袭络、浊气上冲巧坞或气血亏损及瘀血内阻，导致三道两路闭阻，巧坞失其濡养，发为巧尹。其主要的发病机理如下。

The onset of "Qiaoyin" is related to external contraction of wind, cold and/or dampness as well as injury to the liver, spleen and/or kidney. When pathogenic wind attacks the collaterals, turbid qi enters the head, blood and qi are deficient and/or blood stasis stagnates in the body, the three passages and two channels will be blocked. This will cause the head to lack nutrients, resulting in headache. There are four types of mechanism.

（1）外感风湿、痧瘴、蛊毒。起居不慎，感受风湿、痧瘴、蛊毒之邪，邪气上犯巅顶，侵扰巧坞，导致巧坞不通而发病。

(1) External contraction of wind-dampness, miasma of filth and/or parasitic toxin, and irregular life causes the body to be attacked by the pathogenic qi derived from wind-dampness, miasma of filth and/or parasitic toxin. When ascending to the head, the pathogenic qi will block the head, leading to headache.

（2）情志失调。忧郁恼怒，情志不遂，肝失条达，气郁阳亢，或肝郁化火，阳亢火生，上扰巧坞而发病。

(2) Excess emotional activity such as depression and irritation impair the free flow of liver qi. This will results in qi depression and ascendant hyperactivity of liver yang. It can also cause liver depression transforming into fire and hyperactivity of liver yang transforming into fire. Consequently, the head is affected, leading to headache.

（3）饮食劳倦。饮食所伤，劳逸失度，脾失健运，痰湿内生，使清阳不升，浊阴不降，巧坞痹阻而发病。

(3) Improper diet and overstrain, injury due to diet, imbalance between work and rest and/or dysfunction of the spleen in transportation lead to internal dampness-phlegm, and cause clear yang qi not to ascend and turbid qi not to descend. Consequently, the head is blocked, leading to headache.

（4）先天不足或体虚久病。先天不足，或病后、产后、失血之后，营血亏损，脑髓失充，巧坞失养而发病。

(4) Congenital defect, weak constitution due to chronic illness and/or reduction of nutrient blood after illness, childbirth, blood loss cause insufficiency of brain marrow. Consequently, the head does not have adequate nourishment, leading to headache.

3. 诊察要点

3.3　Essentials for diagnosis

（1）诊断依据。

(1) Diagnosis criteria.

① 主症：头部胀痛、刺痛、钝痛或灼痛，或阵作，或持续。

① Main symptoms: Headache may be manifested as a distending pain, a stabbing pain, a dull pain and a burning pain, which are persistent or intermittent.

②兼症：面红目赤，烦躁易怒，口苦梦多，面部颜色呈青色或黑色，舌质红或暗紫，呈瘀斑舌，舌下脉络粗胀，腰膝酸软，耳鸣少寐，神疲乏力，脸色无华等。

② Concurrent symptoms: Reddened complexion with crimson eyes, vexation, irritability, bitter taste in the mouth, profuse dreaming, bluish or black complexion without luster, reddish or dark purple tongue with ecchymosis, dilated blood vessels under the tongue, soreness and weakness in the lumbar region and knees, tinnitus, less sleep, lassitude.

③目诊。勒答上白睛脉络弯曲少，弯度小，颜色浅。

③ Eye examination: The blood vessels on the white of the eyes are reddish with a few small-radius bends.

④甲诊。指甲颜色深红或鲜红，半月痕暴露过多，呈紫赤甲或横沟甲。

④ Nail examination: Dark or bright red fingernails with large fingernail lunulae. There are red-purple dots or Beau's lines on nail beds.

（2）病证鉴别。

(2) Symptom differentiation.

①眩晕。眩晕以头晕眼花为主要临床表现，轻者闭目可止，重者如坐舟船，旋转不定，不能站立，或伴有头痛、恶心、呕吐、汗出、面色苍白等症状。而巧尹主要以头部疼痛为主症，一侧、双侧或全头疼痛，呈跳痛、胀痛、刺痛等，无头晕眼花，无视物旋转，故可相区别。

① Dizziness: The main clinical manifestations are lightheadness and blurred vision. Light dizziness disappears when the eyes are closed. With severe dizziness, the person has the false sense that either the environment or one's own body is revolving, like on a boat. They cannot stand up and may have other symptoms such as headache, nausea, vomiting, sweating or pale complexion. On the other hand, headache may be manifested as a throbbing pain, a distending pain and a stabbing pain on one or two sides of the head or across the head. Patients with headache do not feel lightheaded or have spatial disorientation.

②真头痛。真头痛多为突然剧烈头痛，常表现为持续痛而阵发加重，甚则伴喷射性呕吐、肢厥、抽搐等。

② True headache: A critical case of headache marked by sudden attack of pain in the head. Normally, the pain is persistent, but if it is intermittent, it will become worse, which may be accompanied by projectile vomiting, cold extremities and convulsions.

③ 中风。中风以猝然昏仆、不省人事、口舌歪斜、半身不遂、失语等为主要症状。也有部分中风病人以头痛、眩晕为先兆表现。巧尹以头痛为主，无眩晕、猝然昏仆、不省人事等表现，故可相区别。

③ Wind stroke: A disease characterized by sudden loss of consciousness, distortion of the mouth and tongue, sudden appearance of hemiplegia and impeded speech. For some patients, wind stroke is preceded by headache and lightheadedness. On the other hand, patients with headache do not experience lightheadedness or sudden loss of consciousness.

④ 不寐。轻者表现为入睡困难，或寐而不酣、时寐时醒，或醒后不能再寐；重者则彻夜不寐。常伴有头痛、头昏、心悸、神疲乏力等症状。巧尹患者头痛呈昏沉感，虽有睡眠欠佳症状，但均在头痛时发作，故可相区别。

④ Insomnia: People with slight insomnia have difficulty falling asleep or staying asleep. They experience mid-sleep awakening or cannot fall asleep again after waking up. People with severe insomnia are sleepless through the night. Insomnia is often accompanied by headache, lightheadedness, palpitation and/or lassitude of spirit. In contrast, patients with headache are normally drowsy and unable to sleep well, but such symptoms only occur during the headache attack.

4. 辨证论治

3.4　Syndrome differentiation and treatment

（1）治疗原则。调气补虚，通路止痛。

(1) Treatment principles. To adjust qi and reinforce deficiency and unblock two channels to relieve pain.

（2）证治分类。

(2) Classification of syndrome identification and treatment.

① 主穴。风池、太阳、率谷及 3 个壮医特定穴食魁、中魁和无魁（分别位于食指、中指和无名指近端指间关节中点上 5 分处）、梅花穴（在痛处取之）。

① Primary acupoints: Fengchi (GB 20), Taiyang (EX-HN 5), Shuaigu (GB 8), three points respectively on the dorsal side of the index finger, middle finger and ring finger, at the center of the proximal interphalangeal joint[*], and a point in the tender spot with other points on its corner, which looks like a plum flower.

② 辨证分型选穴。

② Acupoints selection after syndrome differentiation.

阳证。

Yang syndrome.

若为风热头痛，则主症：头痛而胀，甚则头痛如裂，发热或恶风，面红目赤，口渴欲饮，便秘，舌红苔黄，脉浮数。

Wind-heat headache: Distending pain, or even splitting pain in the head, fever, aversion to cold, reddened complexion with crimson eyes, thirst with desire to drink, constipation, red tongue with yellow coating and floating, rapid pulse.

取穴：梅花穴、风池、太阳、率谷、丝竹空、大椎、合谷、列缺、曲池。

Acupoints selection: A point in the affected area with other points on its corner, which looks like a plum flower, Fengchi (GB 20), Taiyang (EX-HN 5), Shuaigu (GB 8), Sizhukong (TE 23), Dazhui (GV 14), Hegu (LI 4), Lieque (LU 7) and Quchi (LI 11).

若为风湿头痛，则主症：头痛如裹，肢体困重，纳呆胸闷，小便不利，大便溏烂，苔白腻，脉濡。

Wind-dampness headache: Headache with a feeling that the head is tightly wrapped, heavy sensation in the limbs, chest stuffiness, dysuria, loose stools, white and greasy tongue coating, soggy pulse.

取穴：梅花穴、风池、太阳、率谷、印堂、中脘、丰隆。

Acupoints selection: A point in the affected area with other points on its corner, which looks like a plum flower, Fengchi (GB 20), Taiyang (EX-HN 5), Shuaigu (GB 8), Yintang (EX-HN 3), Zhongwan (CV 12) and Fenglong (ST 40).

若为肝阳头痛，则主症：头痛而眩，心烦易怒，夜眠不宁，或兼胁痛，面

---

* These three points are uniquely used in Zhuang medicine.

红口苦，舌苔薄黄，脉弦有力。

Liver-yang headache: Pain in the head with dizziness which may be accompanied by hypochondriac pain, vexation, irritability, dream-disturbed sleep, reddened complexion, bitter taste in the mouth, yellow and thin tongue coating, and wiry, forceful pulse.

取穴：梅花穴、风池、太阳、率谷、头维、上星、行间、太冲、太溪。

Acupoints selection: A point in the affected area with other points on its corner, which looks like a plum flower, Fengchi (GB 20), Taiyang (EX-HN 5), Shuaigu (GB 8), Touwei (ST 8), Shangxing (DU 23), Xingjian (LR 2), Taichong (LR 3) and Taixi (KI 3).

若为痰浊头痛，则主症：头痛昏蒙，胸脘满闷，呕恶痰涎，苔白腻，脉滑或弦滑。

Phlegm-turbidity headache: Pain in the head and mental confusion, chest stuffiness, nausea, expectoration, white and greasy tongue coating, slippery or wiry pulse.

取穴：梅花穴、风池、太阳、率谷、印堂、中脘、丰隆。

Acupoints selection: A point in the affected area with other points on its corner, which looks like a plum flower, Fengchi (GB 20), Taiyang (EX-HN 5), Shuaigu (GB 8), Yintang (EX-HN 3), Zhongwan (CV 12) and Fenglong (ST 40).

阴证。

Yin syndrome.

若为风寒头痛，则主症：头痛时作，痛连项背，遇风尤剧，恶风畏寒，口不渴，舌苔薄白，脉浮。

Wind-cold headache: Pain in the head which extends to the nape and back is worsened by wind, aversion to wind, intolerance of cold, absence of thirst, white and thin tongue coating, floating pulse.

取穴：梅花穴、风池、太阳、率谷、百会、手三里、合谷。

Acupoints selection: A point in the affected area with other points on its corner, which looks like a plum flower, Fengchi (GB 20), Taiyang (EX-HN 5), Shuaigu (GB 8), Baihui (DU 20), Shousanli (LI 13) and Hegu (LI 4).

若为肾虚头痛，则主症：头痛且空，每兼眩晕，腰痛酸软，神疲乏力，遗精带下，耳鸣少寐，舌红苔少，脉细。

Kidney-insufficiency headache: Empty pain in the head with dizziness, lumbar aching, lassitude of spirit, seminal emission or vaginal discharge, tinnitus, less sleep, red tongue with a little coating, thready pulse.

取穴：梅花穴、风池、太阳、率谷、肾俞、肝俞、照海。

Acupoints selection: A point in the affected area with other points on its corner, which looks like a plum flower, Fengchi (GB 20), Taiyang (EX-HN 5), Shuaigu (GB 8), Shenshu (BL 23), Ganshu (BL 18) and Zhaohai (KI 6).

若为血虚头痛，则主症：头痛而晕，心悸不宁，神疲乏力，面色苍白，舌质淡，苔薄白，脉细弱。

Blood-deficiency headache: Pain in the head with dizziness, palpitation, lassitude of spirit, pale complexion, pale tongue with white, thin coating, thready and weak pulse.

取穴：梅花穴、风池、太阳、率谷、上星、三阴交、足三里、血海。

Acupoints selection: A point in the affected area with other points on its corner, which looks like a plum flower, Fengchi (GB 20), Taiyang (EX-HN 5), Shuaigu (GB 8), Shangxing (DU 23), Sanyinjiao (SP 6), Zusanli (ST 36) and Xuehai (SP 10).

若为瘀血头痛，则主症：头痛经久不愈，痛处固定不移，痛如锥刺，或有头部外伤史，舌质紫，苔薄白，脉细或细涩。

Blood-stasis headache: Refractory stabbing and fixed pain in the head, which may occur after traumatic injury, purple tongue with white, thin coating, and thready or thready, choppy pulse.

取穴：梅花穴、风池、太阳、率谷、内关、血海、膈俞。

Acupoints selection: A point in the affected area with other points on its corner, which looks like a plum flower, Fengchi (GB 20), Taiyang (EX-HN 5), Shuaigu (GB 8), Neiguan (PC 6), Xuehai (SP 10) and Geshu (BL 17).

5. 预防调护

3.5　Prevention and care

（1）本法对神经功能性头痛疗效较好，对头颅部实质性病变者疗效欠佳，应明确诊断，正确治疗。

(1) The ZM medicated thread moxibustion has remarkable efficacy on neurological headaches but poor efficacy on brain lesions, so before treatment, syndromes should be differentiated.

（2）可结合做头面部的穴位保健按摩，或常梳理头皮，刺激头部血液循环。

(2) Massage on the head and face, or often comb the scalp to stimulate blood circulation in the head.

（3）舒畅情志，保证充分睡眠和适当休息。保持平常心态，注意饮食卫生。

(3) Maintain a healthy relationship with emotions, ensure adequate sleep and proper rest, keep a peaceful mind and have a clean diet.

6. 医案选读

3.6　Selected case readings

【病案一】

［Case 1］

王某，女，39 岁，2020 年 10 月 2 日就诊。

Patient: Wang, a 39-year-old woman; her first visit was on October 2, 2020.

主诉：左侧偏头痛 2 年余，多在劳累及睡眠欠佳时诱发，发作时感左太阳穴处跳痛，渐扩展至整个半侧头部，每次发作历时数小时至数日不等。夜不能眠。此次复发，在外院治疗，效果甚微。

Chief complaint:"I have had migraine on the left side of my head for more than 2 years. It often happened due to exertion or lack of sleep. Throbbing pain started in my left temple, which gradually radiated across the left side of my head. It could last for a few hours or a few days, resulting in sleeplessness. I had treatment at other hospital this time but it was not effective."

查体：痛苦病容，血压 142/87 mmHg，心率 92 次 / 分，律齐，肺部正常。舌淡红，苔薄白，脉弦数。

Physical examination: The patient has a painful morbid complexion. Her blood pressure (BP) is 142/87 mmHg. She has a normal sinus rhythm with a heart rate of 92 beats/min. Her lungs are normal. Her tongue is light red with white, thick coating. Her pulse is thready and rapid.

壮医诊断：巧尹（阳证）。中医诊断：头痛（肝阳头痛）。西医诊断：血管神经性头痛。

Diagnosis in ZM:"Qiaoyin", characterized by yang syndrome.

Diagnosis in TCM: Liver-yang headache.

Diagnosis in WM: Angioneurotic headache.

取穴：攒竹、头维、右侧食魁（左侧头痛取对侧穴位）、太阳，每穴 2 壮，每日 1 次。灸治当天，头部跳痛明显减轻，当夜安睡，次日灸后头痛痊愈，继续巩固灸治 2 日。

Acupoints selection: Cuanzhu (BL 2), Touwei (ST 8), point on the dorsal side of the right index finger, at the center of the proximal interphalangeal joint (selecting the point on the right side for treating migraine occurring on the left side) and Taiyang (EX-HN 5). Two cones were applied to each point, one time of treatment daily. On the first day, the throbbing pain was significantly relieved, which made her sleep well that night. It disappeared after treatment on the second day. Then, the moxibustion was applied another 2 days to consolidate the efficacy.

【病案二】

［Case 2］

郭某，女，40 岁，2019 年 8 月 20 日初诊。

Patient: Guo, a 40-year-old woman; her first visit was on August 20, 2019.

主诉：头痛 1 周，以左侧及巅顶尤甚，伴恶寒反复发作。月经 2 日前净。

Chief complaint:"I have had pain in my head for one week, especially on the left side and at the top of my head. I had aversion to cold which was recurrent. My menstruation ended 2 days ago."

查体：脉沉细，舌淡，苔薄白。

Physical examination: Her pulse is deep and thready. Her tongue is pale with white, thin coating.

壮医诊断：巧尹（阴证）。中医诊断：头痛（血虚型）。西医诊断：经后期头痛。

Diagnosis in ZM:"Qiaoyin", characterized by yin syndrome.

Diagnosis in TCM: Blood-deficiency headache.

Diagnosis in WM: Postmenstrual headache.

治疗原则：补气血，祛风止痛。

Treatment principles: Tonify qi and blood, dispel wind and relieve pain.

取穴：阿是穴、百会、四神聪、风池、印堂、太阳、合谷、足三里、关元，连续点灸 4 次而愈（图 14、图 15）。

Acupoints selection: Ashi points, Baihui (DU 20), Sishencong (EX-HN-1), Fengchi (GB 20), Yintang (EX-HN 3), Taiyang (EX-HN 5), Hegu (LI 4), Zusanli (ST 36) and Guanyuan (CV 4). The pain disappeared after the patient had the treatment 4 times (Fig. 14 and Fig. 15).

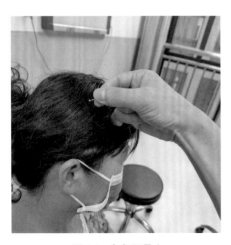 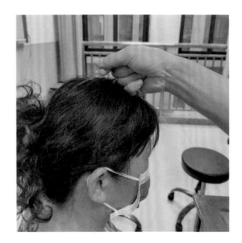

图 14　点灸阿是穴 | 图 15　点灸百会穴
Fig. 14　Moxibustion on a Ashi point | Fig. 15　Moxibustion on Baihui

按语：患者经后头痛为营血亏虚，不能上荣于脑髓脉络而致，既往反复发作。风气久客，头为诸阳之会，手足三阳经脉均循头面，用百会、四神聪能防风止痛，脉沉细、舌淡、苔薄白均为气血亏虚之象，用合谷补气血，足三里健运脾胃，灸印堂、太阳、风池等局部穴位而愈，诸穴起调气补虚、通路止痛的作用。

Summary statement: The patient's postmenstrual headache was caused by insufficiency of nutrient blood which was unable to flow upward to the blood vessels in the head. Such disorder recurred, resulting in stagnation of pathological wind in the head where all the yang meridians/channels meet. Since the three yang meridians/channels of the hand and the feet go through the face and meet in the head, moxibustion on Baihui (GV 20) and Sishencong (EX-HN 1) can prevent the attack of wind and relieve pain. Her deep, thready pulse and pale tongue with white, thin coating were the signs of insufficiency of qi and blood, so Hegu (LI 4) was used to tonify qi and blood, Zusanli (ST 36) was used to invigorate the spleen and stomach, and Yintang (EX-HN 3) combined with Taiyang (EX-HN 5) and Fengchi (GB 20) were used to make the pain disappear. Moxibustion on all these points can adjust qi, reinforce deficiency and unblock the channels to relieve pain.

第三章　壮医脐环穴针刺疗法

Chapter 3　Acupuncture at the Umbilical Ring Point in Zhuang Medicine

一、疗法概况

Ⅰ　Introduction

（一）发展历史

1　History of the acupuncture at the umbilical ring point in Zhuang medicine

中医针灸经典名著《针灸甲乙经》中提到："脐中禁不可刺。"但壮医对脐有着独特的认识。古壮医对脐的解剖认识基于古代壮族人民对尸体解剖的认识。北宋庆历年间，在壮族人民聚居的广西宜州发生了一起农民起义，统治阶级抓捕并处死了欧希范等起义首领56人，随后命宜州推官吴简、绘工宋景及医官等人对全部尸体进行解剖，绘成图谱，命名为《欧希范五脏图》。该图谱所绘内容主要为人体内脏结构，对肝、肾、心、胞宫、大网膜等器官结构做了详细记载。该图谱是我国医学史上第一张实绘人体解剖图，对加深壮医在人体解剖及生理方面的认识具有很大的促进作用。

A-B Classic of Acupuncture and Moxibustion, a classic TCM book, states that "The umbilicus is forbidden to be needled". However, there is a unique understanding of the umbilicus in Zhuang medicine (ZM), based on the ancient Zhuang nationality's anatomical knowledge. Ou Xifan and other fifty-five leaders of the peasant uprising, which started in Yizhou, Guangxi, a region for the Zhuang people, in 1044 (the 4th year of Qingli in the Northern Song Dynasty), were killed by the ruling class. Then, their corpses were dissected by authorized doctors with the participation of Wu Jian, a judicial official, and Song Jing, a painter. Based on sketches of the organs of those executed rebel fighters, *Ou Xifan's Diagrams of the Five Organs* was created. As the first anatomical atlas in the history of Chinese medicine, it mainly illustrates human internal organs, including the anatomical positions and shapes of the liver, kidney, heart, uterus and omentum. It greatly helped ZM practitioners to understand the structure and physiology of the human body.

壮医不但认为脐可以灸，还将脐作为常规的针灸穴位。例如1934年出任广西省立南宁区医药研究所所长的刘惠宁先生（字六桥，号潜初，前国医馆理事，国医大师班秀文教授的老师）的著作《六桥医话》中，就有这样的记载："尝见一童子患风搐，一妇人教捉竹丝鸡置尾敷于童子脐上，鸡则自用力坐实，放手逐之不去，似甚畅美，不能相舍之状，又似电之相吸者然，少顷童子抽搐不作，而鸡去矣。"

From the perspective of ZM, points on the umbilicus can be used as conventional acupoints for moxibustion and acupuncture. *Lectures of Liuqiao medicine* written by Liu Huining* describes a scene: When infantile convulsions occurred in a child, a woman put the tail of a white-feathered chicken with dark skin on the child's umbilicus. The chicken firmly sat on its own and its feet firmly held the child's belly, which looked like the attraction of opposite charges. After a while, infantile convulsions seizure disappeared and the chicken left.

脐穴在壮族民间流传很广，现存第一部以壮医命名的著作《壮医药线点灸疗法》中就有"脐周四穴"的描述。到20世纪80年代，壮医临床奠基人、国家级非物质文化遗产壮医药线点灸疗法传承人、全国名老中医黄瑾明教授带领团队深入壮族民间，挖掘整理壮医肚脐疗法并进行临床观察验证，逐渐整理出一套壮医脐环穴理论体系，并在其编著的第一部壮医针灸专著《中国壮医针灸学》中第一次明确提出脐环穴穴名。黄瑾明还将针灸脐环穴作为临床治疗各科疾病的首选手段，治愈了大量患者。

The umbilical ring point is widely known among the Zhuang people. The description of it is as early as in the first existing book about Zhuang medicine, *The Zhuang Medicine Medicated Thread Moxibustion*. In the 1980s, a set of theories

---

* Liu Huining, whose style name is "Liuqiao" and pseudonym is "Qianchu", started work as a director of at the Medical Research Institute of Nanning, Guangxi in 1934, and afterwards, became the director of the National Medical Center and the teacher of Professor Ban Xiuwen who is also a TCM master.

about it were established by Huang Jinming* and his team after they had collated all information about the therapy and conducted clinical observation and verification. The umbilical ring points were first clearly stated in *China's Zhuang Medicine Acupuncture* edited by Huang Jinming. He considered needling these points as a preferred treatment method in his medical practice and cured many patients.

（二）治疗机理

2　Treatment mechanism

壮医认为，脐是体内道路系统的一个特殊网结，与全身各脏腑组织有着密切的联系，是人整体的缩影，人体各脏腑器官在脐部的投影犹如一个正立位的胎儿，其投影的位置与人体脏器的正常位置相对应（图 16）。

From the perspective of ZM, as a special node of the network formed by the passages and channels, the umbilicus is closely correlated to zang-fu organs and can be considered as the epitome of the body. The image formed by the projection of all organs on the umbilicus is like a fetus in an upright position. The position of each organ in the projected image corresponds to its normal position in the body (Fig. 16).

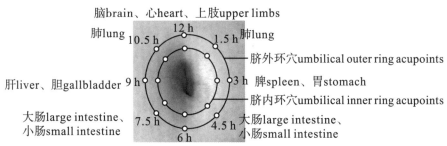

脑brain、心heart、上肢upper limbs
肺lung　12 h　肺lung
10.5 h　1.5 h
脐外环穴umbilical outer ring acupoints
肝liver、胆gallbladder　9 h　3 h　脾spleen、胃stomach
脐内环穴umbilical inner ring acupoints
大肠large intestine、　7.5 h　4.5 h　大肠large intestine、
小肠small intestine　6 h　小肠small intestine
肾kidney、膀胱bladder、胞宫womb、卵巢oarium、
睾丸testicle、前列腺prostate、下肢lower limbs

图 16　脐环穴与脏腑对应图

Fig. 16　A correspondence map of umbilical ring acupoints and the zang-fu organs

壮医在长期的临床实践中逐渐认识到，龙路、火路是人体内部的两条极为

---

* Huang Jinming, a nationally well-known TCM practitioner and professor of Guangxi University of Chinese Medicine. He is considered as a father of ZM practices and designated as the representative inheritor of the ZM medicated thread moxibustion inscribed on the Representative List of State-level Intangible Cultural Heritage of Humanity.

重要的通道，龙路的中枢在咪心头（心），火路的中枢在巧坞，龙路、火路均有干线和网络，其内有气血运行，循环往来，如环无端。龙路主运行气血，营养全身；火路主传感信息，即时做出反应。龙路、火路的分支遍布全身，它们内属脏腑，外络肢节，沟通三道，贯通上下左右，再加上谷道、水道、气道的沟通联系，将内部的脏腑骨肉同外部的各种组织官窍及人体的天部、地部、人部联结成为一个有机的整体，使人体各部的气血保持相对的调畅平衡，各部功能得以正常发挥，人体处于健康状态。

In the long-term practices of ZM, the following thoughts have developed: The dragon and fire channels are extremely important paths in the human body; the heart ("Mixintou" in the Zhuang language) is the center of the dragon channel while the brain ("Qiaowu" in the Zhuang language) is the center of the fire channel; the two channels consist of main and branch lines, forming a cycle, in which qi and blood circulate; nutrients are transported throughout the body by the movement of qi and blood in the dragon channel while the fire channel functions like a sensor reacting to the environment; and as part of zang-fu organs, these two channels running through the body make tissues and other organs connected. They are also associated with the grain, water and qi passages. Thus, internal organs, bones, muscles, orifices of sense organs, and the heaven, earth and human parts of the body are connected into an organic whole. Consequently, qi and blood in all parts of the body move smoothly and coordinate, and the organs work properly. This ensures the body remains healthy.

道路系统是壮医脐环穴针刺疗法应用的理论基础。龙路、火路在人体体表密布其网络分支，这些分支在人体体表一定部位交叉成结，壮医称之为网结，又称穴位，是人体气血交汇结聚之处，人体体表有很多这样的网结。谷道、水道、气道虽然在人体体表没有网络分支，但在人体体表一定部位常存在反应点，壮医把这些反应点也称为穴位，又称压痛点或敏感点。因此，三道两路在人体体表均有穴位分布，刺激这些穴位就可以作用于相应的道路及脏腑。壮医脐环穴针刺疗法，就是在脐周各穴位施以针刺治疗，通过龙路、火路的传导，畅通三道两路系统，一方面调节、激发或通畅人体之气血，损其偏胜，补其偏衰，使之正常运行，趋于均衡，与天、地之气保持同步；另一方面增强正气，提高人体抗病能力，加速邪毒化解或通过三道排出体外，使天、地、人三部之气复归同步，进而使疾病痊愈。

According to the theory of three passages and two channels, branch lines of the dragon and fire channels along the body superficies intersect at many places. These intersections, also known as nodes or acupoints in ZM, are where qi and blood converge. Although there are no branch lines of the grain, water and qi passages on the body superficies, there are their reaction points, which are considered as acupoints in ZM and are called points of tenderness or sensitivity. Therefore, stimulating all these points can regulate the functions of the passages, channels and organs. The above theory provides a basis for the application of acupuncture at the umbilical ring point in ZM. In this therapeutic method, needling the acupoints around the umbilicus can unblock the three passages and two channels through the conduction of the dragon and fire channels. Thus, qi and blood are adjusted, stimulated or moved to neutralize abnormal exuberance or deficiency of qi and blood, leading to their harmony. Also, the healthy qi is strengthened, the body's natural defenses are boosted and toxins are more quickly resolved or drawn out through the three passages. Consequently, the heaven-qi, earth-qi and the human-qi can be synchronized, resulting in a cure of disease.

由此可见，脐相当于人体的"微诊系统"，像勒答、耳朵、指甲等一样，是人体的缩影，在疾病诊断上具有特殊的定性定位和预后价值，通过观脐可以察知人体的健康状况；脐同时又是一个治疗全身疾病的窗口，刺激此窗口的相应位置，就能通过道路系统的传导，作用于相应的组织器官，从而治疗全身疾病。

Therefore, as a micro-diagnosis system of the human body and the epitome of the human body like the eyes, ears and nails, the umbilicus can be observed to learn about the body's health. This can help to determine the nature and location of a disease and has prognostic value. Also, different sites of the umbilicus can be stimulated to regulate the functions of the corresponding organs through the conduction of the passages and channels, enabling diseases occurring at any part of the body to be cured.

（三）主要功效

3　Main efficacy

根据临床实践总结和实验研究结果，壮医脐环穴针刺疗法具有以下主要功效。

Experience from clinical practice and results from experimental research show the following efficacy of the acupuncture at the umbilical ring point in ZM.

1. 通畅道路，活血祛毒

3.1　To unblock the passages and channels, activate blood and remove toxins

壮医脐环穴针刺疗法有通调道路、活血祛毒的作用。通过对穴位的针刺刺激，可以祛瘀消滞、畅通三道、调达两路，使三道两路畅通而发挥其正常的生理功能，使天、地、人三气恢复同步功能。这是壮医脐环穴针刺疗法最基本和最直接的作用。

The most basic and direct therapeutic effectiveness of acupuncture at the umbilical ring point in ZM is to regulate the passages and channels, activate blood and remove toxins. In other words, stimulating points on the umbilicus with needles removes blood stasis and qi stagnation so as to unblock the three passages and the two channels. This will ensure these passages and channels to perform their own normal physiological functions, resulting in the restoration of synchronization of the heaven-qi, earth-qi and human-qi.

壮医认为，三道两路以通为用，以塞为痛，以阻为病。三道畅通，调节有度，人体之气就能与天地之气保持同步协调平衡；三道阻塞或调节失度，则天、地、人三气不能同步而产生各种病痛；龙路受阻，则无法为脏腑、骨肉输送营养；火路阻断，则人体失去对外界信息的反应、适应能力，以致发生各种疾病甚至死亡。塞和阻来自瘀、滞，或虚弱、两路不足而致连接不通。穴位是人体三道两路运行气血的出入之处，是脏腑、气血、骨肉之外延，是天、地、人三部运行气血的重要通道，是三道两路在人体体表布设的网结。针刺通过刺激脐周穴位并迅速传导至巧坞令其立即作出反应，调动体内之壮气使三道两路畅通，或通过濡养，补充不足，使两路能连接畅通，祛毒外出，使三气归于同步。

From the perspective of ZM, free flow in the three passages and two channels maintain their functions, but stagnation in them causes pain and blockage of them leads to diseases. Specifically, if the passages and channels are smooth and coordinated, the human-qi can be synchronized with the heaven-qi and earth-qi. On the other hand, if they are blocked or uncoordinated, these three kinds of qi will fail to keep pace with each other, resulting in diseases. Blockage of the dragon channel makes nutrients fail to be transported to zang-fu organs, bones and muscles while interrupted fire channel makes the human body unable to respond and adapt to the environment. As a result, diseases occur, of which some may lead to death. "Blo-ckage" and "interruption" are caused by stasis and stagnation, or the deficiency of the two channels due to weak constitution. Acupoints are the places at which qi and blood in the three passages and two channels are regulated and through which qi and blood move in the heaven, earth and human parts of the body. They are extensions of zang-fu organs, qi, blood, muscles and bones, as well as nodes of the network on the body superficies, formed by the three passages and two channels. Therefore, when the points around the umbilicus are stimulated with needles, the brain will respond by mobilizing the healthy qi to unblock the three passages and two channels, or by absorbing nutrients to reinforce deficiency. Thus, the two channels are connected and toxins are drawn out, leading to synchronization of the human-qi, heaven-qi and earth-qi.

2. 均衡气血阴阳

3.2　To balance qi-blood and yin-yang

壮医脐环穴针刺疗法有均衡气血阴阳的作用。针刺可使机体从气血阴阳不均衡状态向平衡状态转化，这是壮医脐环穴针刺治疗最终要达到的目的。通过针刺刺激脐周的穴位，经火路传导，传至巧坞，巧坞能够快速作出反应，迅速激活人体的自愈力，有目的地为机体的调节机制提供援助，帮助机体的内在自愈系统充分地发挥作用，调整气血阴阳恢复平衡，促使疾病向痊愈方向转归，使机体维持健康的状态，从而达到治愈疾病的目的。

The acupuncture at the umbilical ring point in ZM aims to restore the balance of qi-blood and yin-yang. Specifically, when receiving the signals, which are produced by acupuncture at the points around the umbilicus, through the fire channel, the brain will rapidly respond by activating the body's healing ability which can provide assistance as needed to the regulating mechanisms in the body and make the self-healing system work well. Thus, the balance between qi-blood and yin-yang can be restored, promoting recovery from diseases and making the body remain healthy.

3. 调神减压

3.3　To adjust the mind and reduce stress

壮医脐环穴针刺疗法有调神减压的作用。随着现代生活节奏的加快，人们的压力与忙碌同步攀升，来自社会、工作、家庭各方面的压力有时会使大家喘不过气来。面对这些压力，许多人患了忧郁、焦虑、失眠等病证。壮医脐环穴针刺疗法通过针刺人体的脐周穴位，使之产生刺激能量信息并迅速通过火路传至巧坞，巧坞之"神"快速作出反应，调整机体各种机能，有目的地为机体的调节机制提供援助，帮助机体的内在自愈系统充分发挥作用，使机体放松，减缓压力。其治疗的真谛在于调"神"和治"神"。故临床应用于治疗一些情志不舒、心神不宁的疾病，如失眠、忧郁、焦虑、神经官能症、更年期综合征等疾病，能起到良好的治疗效果。

Due to the increasingly rapid pace and complexity of life, people tend to lead a hectic life and have to face the huge pressure from society, work and family. Consequently, some of them suffer from mental and emotional disorders such as depression, anxiety and insomnia. The acupuncture at the umbilical ring point in ZM can be used to adjust the mind and reduce stress. Specifically, when receiving the signals, which are produced by acupuncture on the points around the umbilicus, through the fire channel, the brain will rapidly respond by activating the body's healing ability which can provide assistance as needed to the regulating mechanisms in the body and make the self-healing system work well. Thus, the body can be relaxed and stress will be reduced. The essence of the therapy is to adjust and manage the mind. Therefore, it has remarkable efficacy on the treatment of mental and emotional disorders such as insomnia, depression, anxiety, neurosis and menopausal syndrome.

4. 扶正补虚

3.4　To reinforce the healthy qi and tonify deficiency

壮医脐环穴针刺疗法有扶正补虚的作用。壮医认为，疾病产生的过程，就是正邪相争的过程，而能否导致机体产生病变，就看正邪相争谁胜谁负。壮医脐环穴针刺疗法治疗疾病，就是通过针刺对穴位的刺激，扶助正气，激活并增强人体的自愈力，祛除病邪，增加身体的正能量，改变正邪双方的力量比，使正战胜邪，天、地、人三气复归同步，从而促进疾病向痊愈方向转归和人体正气康复，这是扶正补虚的一个方面；而另一方面，对于各种虚弱患者，选择有强壮作用的脐周环穴定期施予针刺，可以匡扶正气，增强体质，激活并增强人体的自愈力，从而达到防病保健、强壮身体的作用。

The acupuncture at the umbilical ring point in ZM can be used to reinforce the healthy qi and tonify deficiency. From the perspective of ZM, the occurrence of any disease is a process of struggle between the healthy qi and pathogenic qi. The exuberance of the pathogenic qi with the debilitation of the healthy qi results in diseases. Needling the points around the umbilicus can reinforce the healthy qi and tonify deficiency, activate and improve the body's healing ability and remove pathogenic qi. This will make the healthy qi rise and the pathogenic qi decline. Consequently, the heaven-qi, earth-qi and human-qi are synchronized, resulting in the improvement of the healthy qi and the recovery from the disease. In addition, for those with weak constitution, the therapy can be used to reinforce the healthy qi to strengthen the body, and activate and improve the body's healing ability, and thereby achieve disease prevention and health promotion.

二、技法特色
Ⅱ Characteristics of the therapy

（一）理论特色
1 Theoretical features

与传统中医针灸不同，壮医针灸明确提出通过壮医道路系统进行传导和调节，以道路学说等理论作为指导思想，而经络学说则没有成为壮医理论基础。

Different from the science of acupuncture and moxibustion of TCM, which is based on the theory of the meridians and collaterals, acupuncture and moxibustion in

ZM are based on the theory of three passages and two channels.

1. 阴阳为本理论

1.1　The yin-yang theory

壮医认为大自然的各种变化都是阴阳对立、阴阳互根、阴阳消长、阴阳平衡、阴阳转化的反应和结果。阴阳为本是"阴阳为本源""阴阳为根本"的意思，阴阳的存在及运动变化都是天地万物运动变化的本源，阴阳的运动变化是天地万物普遍存在的一种客观现象。因此根据壮医阴阳为本理论，人体生理病理的各种变化、各种药物及治疗技法所起的作用、疾病的转归等都是人体内部阴阳运动变化的结果。健康是阴阳协调平衡的结果。

From the perspective of ZM, changes in nature result from opposition, mutual rooting, waxing and waning, balance and conversion of yin and yang. The ceaseless motion of both yin and yang which are opposing and complementing each other—an objective phenomenon, gives rise to all changes seen in the world. Accordingly, the motion of yin and yang of the human body results in physiological and pathological changes in the human body, curative effects of drugs and treatment techniques, and conversion of diseases. Yin-yang harmony guarantees health.

2. 三气同步理论

1.2　The theory of synchronization of the heaven-qi, earth-qi and human-qi

壮医认为，人体的每一部分，都是天、地、人的整体信息的缩影，而脐是体内道路系统的一个特殊网结，与全身各脏腑组织有着密切的联系，是人整体的一个缩影，人体各脏腑器官在脐部的投影犹如一个正立位的胎儿，其投影的位置与人体脏器的正常位置相对应。

From the perspective of ZM, every part of the human body contains the information about heaven, earth and itself. The umbilicus, a special node of the network formed by the passages and the channels, is closely correlated to zang-fu organs. It is the epitome of the body. The image formed by the projection of all organs on the umbilicus is like a fetus in an upright position. The position of each organ in the projected image corresponds to its normal position in the body.

脐处于连接人体人部和地部的枢纽位置，是天部之精气下降及地部之津液上升的路径，脐气正常则天气下降、地气上升、人气调和，从而气血均衡，人体安康。故脐关系到天气的下降、地气的上升及人气的调和，是天、地、人三气的精华所在。把脐部分为天、人、地三部，脐水平线以上为天部；脐水平线为人部；脐水平线以下为地部。天、人、地三部分别与不同的脏腑器官组织相对应。

As a hub, the umbilicus connects the upper body (heaven) to the lower body (earth). Through it, essential qi in the upper body descends while body fluids in the lower body ascend. As the place where the heaven-qi, earth-qi and human-qi converge, the umbilicus is related to the descent of the heaven-qi, the ascent of the earth-qi and the harmony of the human-qi. In other words, if qi in the umbilicus is normal, these three kinds of qi will be harmonized, leading to the balance between qi and blood. This will maintain the body's health. A horizontal line crossing the center of the umbilicus divides the umbilical area into three parts: above the line is heaven, around the line is human and below the line is earth. These three parts correspond to different zang-fu organs.

因此，脐在壮医临床治疗上占有重要位置，人体精气之盛衰，入侵毒邪之浅重，全身的病理变化，皆可通过脐部及脐周察而得之，而脐部的正常与否直接影响到人体生理功能能否正常运行。壮医脐环穴针刺疗法通过道路的传导，一方面调节、激发或通畅人体气血，使之均衡调畅；另一方面增强正气，提高抗病能力，加速邪毒化解或排出体外，使天、地、人三部之气复归同步，从而使疾病痊愈。

Therefore, the umbilicus is valued in ZM practices. By observing it and its surroundings, changes in essential qi, amount of external pathogenic qi and pathological conditions of the body can be learned about. The umbilicus also directly affects human body's physiological function. Acupuncture at the umbilical ring can adjust, stimulate or move qi and blood, resulting in their harmony. It can also strengthen the healthy qi, boost the body's natural defenses and expedite resolving or drawing out toxins, resulting in restoration of synchronization of the heaven-qi, earth-qi and human-qi. Thus, diseases can be cured.

3. 三道两路理论

1.3　The theory of three passages and two channels

从道路理论看，脐周密布龙路、火路的网络分支，位置较浅而显露于外，脐部则是龙路、火路的一个特殊网结，先天时连通花肠、连接母胎，后天时连通谷道，连接咪隆（脾）、咪胴（胃），谷道又是水谷被消化吸收后化生成为人体所需气血的场所，故脐与人体气血密切相关，三道两路之精气皆注于脐。刺激脐部一定位置，可通过龙路、火路等道路系统的传导，调节相应的脏腑器官组织。

According to the theory of three passages and two channels, branch lines of the dragon and fire channels are distributed at shallow depths around the umbilicus. The umbilicus is a specific node of the network formed by these two channels. It connects the uterus to the fetus before birth and the grain passage to the spleen ("Milong" in the Zhuang language) and the stomach ("Midong" in the Zhuang language) after birth. The grain passage is the place where food is digested and absorbed, and then transformed into qi and blood needed by the body. Therefore, the umbilicus is closely related to qi and blood. It is a place where essential qi of the three passages and two channels converge. The signals produced by acupuncture on the points around the umbilicus are transmitted through the dragon and fire channels to regulate the corresponding zang-fu organs.

（二）临床特色

2　Clinical features

1. 适应证范围广

2.1　A wide range of indications

壮医脐环穴针刺疗法适应范围广泛，临床上可以治疗风、寒、湿、痰、瘀等导致三道两路不通、机体平衡失调所引起的痧、瘴、蛊、毒及气道、谷道、水道、龙路、火路的虚证等疾病。

Pathogenic factors such as wind, cold, dampness, phlegm and blood stasis can make the three passages and two channels blocked and the body in imbalance. As a result, filth, miasma, parasite, toxins, and the deficiency of the three passages and two channels will occur, leading to diseases. The acupuncture at the umbilical ring point in ZM can be used to treat these diseases.

2. 疗效显著、起效快

2.2　Remarkable and quick efficacy

壮医脐环穴针刺疗法的临床疗效优势非常明显，主要包括3个方面：第一是适应证范围广、起效迅速；第二是疗效显著且治愈后不反弹；第三是疗效互补的强强联合优势。壮医脐环穴针刺疗法不仅不影响其他疗法和药物治疗的效果，还能与其他疗法和药物互相渗透，相互促进，更有效地提高临床治疗效果。

There are three advantages of the therapy. First, it has a wide range of indications and works quickly. Second, it has remarkable efficacy and can prevent disease recurrence. Third, when it is used with other therapies, it will not affect the efficacy of other therapies or drug treatments, instead, the combined therapies can take synergistic effects to enhance the efficacy of treatment.

3. 安全、无毒副作用

2.3　Safe and free from toxic and side effect

壮医脐环穴针刺疗法不仅无毒无污染，很少有不良反应，而且没有药物带来的毒副作用。壮医脐环穴针刺疗法通过刺激脐环穴实现三道两路的传导和巧坞之"神"的应变，激活和增强了机体的自愈力，使机体的内在自愈系统充分发挥作用，促使疾病转归，是一种绿色的自然疗法，安全可靠，优势明显。

The therapy is free from poison, environmental pollution and toxic effect. When the signals produced by acupuncture on the points around and on the umbilicus are transmitted through the three passages and two channels to the brain which responds quickly, the body's healing ability will be activated and improved. Thus, the human body self-healing system will work well, leading to recovery from diseases. Therefore, the safe and effective therapy is considered as a natural remedy having its own advantages.

4. 治疗成本及费用低廉

2.4　Low cost

壮医脐环穴针刺疗法的经济损耗低，成本及费用相对低廉，能有效降低医疗成本，从根本上解决广大人民群众看病贵、看病难的实际问题，切实减轻人民群众就医费用的负担，符合社会发展和大众需要。

The low cost of the materials used in the therapy results in low-spending treatment, thereby reducing patients' medical bills. This accords with social development and people's needs.

5. 协调治疗作用

2.5 Compatibility

壮医脐环穴针刺疗法可以单独应用，也可以与其他疗法（包括内治法和外治法）联合应用。壮医脐环穴针刺疗法与其他方法联合应用时，不但不影响其他疗法的疗效，而且可以起到疗效协同作用，可提高综合治疗的效果。

The therapy can be used alone or in combination with other therapies. It will not affect the efficacy of other therapies, instead, the combined therapies can take synergistic effects to enhance the efficacy of treatment.

（三）选穴特色

3 Features of acupoints selection

壮医针灸学对脐部有独到的认识，认为脐是人体的缩影，与全身脏腑器官组织相对应，是体内道路系统的一个特殊网结，是全身血脉的汇集点，是天、地、人三部之气交汇的枢纽。在长期的临床实践中，黄瑾明等人逐渐摸索出针灸脐环穴调气的新思路，认为针灸脐环穴的调气作用尤为突出，可疏通三道两路，调节气血均衡，促进三气同步。临床上治疗多种疾病，尤其是内科病时，均喜针灸脐环穴，旨在调气。

As the epitome of the human body, the umbilicus is connected to all internal organs. As a special node of the network formed by the three passages and two channels in the body, it is the place where blood vessels of the whole body intersect and the heaven-qi, earth-qi and human-qi converge. In the long-term ZM practice, Huang Jinming and his team generated new ideas for adjusting qi with the acupuncture at the umbilical points and gained considerable experience. Their clinical experience shows that the greatest advantage of needling the umbilical points is to adjust qi since such treatment can unblock the three passages and two channels, maintain the harmony between qi and blood and help to achieve synchronization of the heaven-qi, earth-qi and human-qi. Therefore, the therapy is a preferred treatment for various diseases, especially internal ones, aiming to adjust qi.

1. 脐内环穴

3.1　Selection of points on the umbilical inner ring

根据脐的形状，在脐窝的外侧缘旁开 0.5 寸（1 寸≈3.33 cm）作一圆环，称脐内环，环线上均是穴位，统称脐内环穴。临床上习惯以钟表位取 8 个穴位，即把脐内环当作一个钟表表盘，以脐中央（神阙）为表盘中心，分别在 12 时、1.5 时、3 时、4.5 时、6 时、7.5 时、9 时、10.5 时 8 个点上取穴，俗称脐内环八穴（图 16）。

In light of the shape of the umbilicus, a circle drawn at a distance of 0.5 cun* from the outer edge of the umbilical fossa is called the inner umbilical ring, on which any point is an acupoint. All of these points are collectively called inner umbilical ring acupoint. Among them, eight points are most often used, which is also known as Eight Umbilical Inner Ring Acupoints. The ring is considered as a clock with Shenque (CV 8) as the center, so these eight points are coded in terms of the 12-hour clock: 12, half past 1, 3, half past 4, 6, half past 7, 9 and half past 10 (Fig. 16).

2. 脐外环穴

3.2　Selection of points on the umbilical outer ring

在脐窝的外侧缘旁开 1.5 寸作一圆环，称脐外环，环线上均是穴位，统称脐外环穴。同样以钟表位取穴，一般取上下左右即 12 时、3 时、6 时、9 时共 4 个穴位，俗称脐周四穴（图 16）。

A circle drawn at a distance of 1.5 cun from the outer edge of the umbilical fossa is called the outer umbilical ring, on which any point is an acupoint. Four points normally selected are coded as 12 o'clock, 3 o'clock, 6 o'clock and 9 o'clock, which is known as Four Umbilical Outer Ring Acupoints (Fig. 16).

---

* Cun is a unit of length for measurement in locating acupoints. 1 cun approximately equal to 3.33 cm. A certain part of the patient's body is divided into certain divisions of equal length, each of which is taken as one proportional unit for measurement.

三、操作规范

Ⅲ　Specifications for operation

（一）前期准备

1　Pre-treatment preparation

1. 治疗环境的准备

1.1　Preparation of the therapeutic environment

治疗室保持整洁，空气新鲜，光线充足，室内温度保持 22 ～ 25 ℃，注意患者保暖。

Keep treatment rooms immaculate, light and airy, and the indoor temperature between 22 ℃ and 25 ℃ , keep the patient warm.

2. 用物准备

1.2　Preparation of materials

治疗盘（垫治疗巾），内盛各种型号的一次性毫针（管针）、复合碘皮肤消毒液、棉签、弯盘、大浴巾、脉枕、一次性利器盒。

Disposable filiform needles with different lengths and gauges, iodopovidone, cotton swabs, a curved tray, large bath towel, pulse performance pillow and disposable sharps container are put into a treatment tray or onto a treatment pad.

需要注意的是，应根据患者的性别、年龄、体形、体质、病情、所选穴位，选取长短、粗细适宜的针具。《灵枢·官针》指出："九针之宜，各有所为，长短大小，各有所施也。"如对于体壮、形胖且病位较深的男性患者，可选取直径 0.3 mm 以上、长度 2 ～ 3 寸的针具；对于体弱、形瘦而病位较浅的女性患者，则应选用直径 0.2 ～ 0.25 mm、长度 1 ～ 2 寸的针具。临床上选择针具，常以将针刺入穴位相应深度，而针身还露在皮肤外少许为宜。

As *Guan Zhen (Official Needling Techniques)* of *Ling Shu (Spiritual Pivot)* points out, nine types of needles varying in length and gauge are used for the treatment of different diseases. Therefore, select needles based on the patient's gender, age, size, constitution, medical conditions and acupoints that will be used. For example, for strong fat man with a disease located deep inside his body, use slightly thicker and longer filiform needles, such as ones with caliber of 0.3 mm or more and length of 2~3 cun; on the other hand, for weak thin women with a disease located superficially, use thinner and shorter filiform needles, such as ones with caliber ranging from 0.2 to 0.25 mm and length of 1~2 cun. Insert needles to various depths at points as appropriate but normally, a part of the needle body remains outside the body.

3. 术前护理

1.3　Pre-acupuncture instructions

（1）核对医嘱，了解患者相关情况，如当前症状、发病部位及相关因素。

(1) Check and explain the acupuncture instructions, understand the patient's medical conditions such as current symptoms, the disease site and the causes of the disease.

（2）做好患者的解释工作。提醒患者针刺过程中如出现头晕、目眩、面色苍白、胸闷、欲呕等症状，属于晕针现象，应及时告知医生。针刺时可能出现疼痛、血肿、滞针、弯针等情况，患者不必紧张，医务人员会妥善处理。如有酸、麻、胀、痛、沉、紧、涩等感觉，属于正常针感。

(2) Advise the patient to make an immediate report if there are symptoms of fainting during acupuncture, including dizziness, blurred vision, pale complexion, chest stuffiness and nausea. Ask them not to be nervous if pain, swelling, sticking of the needle or bending of the needle happens. Tell them a sensation of soreness, numbness, swelling, pain, heaviness, tightness and astringency is normal.

（3）取合理体位（一般取卧位，根据施针穴位所处部位也可以取俯卧位、侧卧位、坐位等），协助患者松开衣着，暴露施术部位以便操作，同时注意患者保暖。

(3) Place the patient in a proper position (normally in the recumbent position, but select the prone, lateral or sitting position if necessary) to make the treatment site exposed and make it convenient for operation. Help the patient to undress but keep them warm.

（二）操作流程

2　Operating procedure

（1）选针。使用 0.25 mm×25 mm 的一次性无菌毫针（1 寸管针）。

(1) Use disposable sterile filiform needles of gauge 0.25 mm × length 25 mm, or with a 25 mm-long fine tube.

（2）取穴。具体方法如前述。

(2) Acupoints selection. The method is the same as described in Paragraph 3 (Features of acupoints selection) of Section Ⅱ.

（3）进针。进针前，嘱患者先做腹式吐纳运动，调整呼吸，平稳情绪，消除紧张感，然后采用管针无痛进针。以脐为中心，向外呈 10° 角放射状平刺，进针深度约为 0.8 寸。

(3) Before needle insertion, instruct the patient to overcome nervousness with diaphragmatic breathing. When their emotions are stabilized, insert needles with fine tube approximately 0.8 cun at an angle of roughly 10 degrees around the umbilicus.

（4）调气方法。进针后嘱患者继续做腹式吐纳运动 3～5 分钟，直至感觉脐部出现暖意。其间，如果患者身体的某个部位出现疼痛或其他不适，提示该处三道两路受阻，需在痛点加刺一针。

(4) After needle insertion, instruct the patient to do diaphragmatic breathing for 3~5 minutes until they have a feeling of warmth in the umbilicus. During treatment, insert a needle in the spot that is indicated by occurrence of pain or discomfort, which means the three passages and two channels are blocked there.

（5）留针。一般留针 30～60 分钟。

(5) Normally retain the needles for 30~60 minutes.

（6）出针。轻柔地将针慢慢拔出。如果针孔出血，立即用消毒棉签按压止血。

(6) Gently withdraw the needles and immediately press the bleeding point with a sterile cotton swab.

（三）注意事项

3　Cautions

（1）向患者做耐心解释，说明壮医针灸主张无痛及在享受中治疗，以消除患者的紧张心理，使其放松心情，配合治疗。

(1) Tell patients that acupuncture and moxibustion in ZM are normally pain-free and comfortable in order to eliminate their nervousness and make them relaxed and cooperative.

（2）严格执行无菌操作。

(2) Strictly implement the aseptic technique procedures.

（3）不宜取站立位治疗，以防患者晕针。

(3) Do not place the patient in the standing position for treatment to prevent fainting.

（4）准确取穴及选择进针方法，掌握好进针角度和深度，勿将针身全部刺入，以防折针。

(4) Find the accurate position of an acupoint and insert a needle at a appropriate depth and angle. Do not insert the needle body completely into the skin to prevent it from breaking.

（5）针刺中应观察患者的面色、神情，询问患者有无不适反应，了解患者心理、生理感受，若发现病情变化立即处理。

(5) During treatment, observe patients' complexion and expression, check whether they are uncomfortable and learn about their psychological and physical feelings. Take corresponding measures if the unexpected happens.

（6）起针时要核对穴位和针数，以免把毫针遗留在患者身上。患者治疗后应避免立即进行剧烈活动。

(6) After needles are withdrawn, check whether the number of punctured acupoints is the same as that of needles inserted to prevent any needles from being left off. After treatment, avoid strenuous activity.

四、常见病证治疗

Ⅳ Treatment of common diseases

（一）核尹（腰痛）

1 Lumbago ("Heyin" in ZM)

1.疾病概述

1.1 General description

核尹指各种原因导致腰部龙路、火路不通，从而出现以腰痛或伴下肢放射痛为主症的病证。相当于中医的腰痹病及西医的腰椎间盘突出症、腰肌劳损、腰椎骨质增生、腰椎退行性病变等引起的腰痛。

Lumbago ("Heyin" in ZM), also known as lumbar impediment in TCM, refers to lower back pain caused by the blockage of the dragon and fire channels in the lumbar region due to different factors. The pain may radiate along the lower limbs. Lumbar diseases in WM, including disc herniation, lumbar muscle strain, vertebral bone hyperplasia and degenerative disease can be included in the domain of "Heyin".

2.病因病机

1.2 Cause and mechanism of disease

核尹发病的主要病因是体虚、气血不足。在三道两路及脏腑功能不足、腰脊虚弱的基础上，外感毒邪，外伤腰部或内伤三道两路、枢纽脏腑，使龙路和火路不通畅，阻滞于腰部，局部龙路、火路功能失调或失养，气血瘀滞于腰府而发为本病。病机多见气血瘀滞，常兼有气血偏衰。

Lumbago occurs mainly due to weak constitution and the deficiency of qi and blood. Specifically, the deficiency of qi and blood in the three passages and two channels, insufficiency of zang-fu organs' functions, and the weakened spine in the lumbar region, which are accompanied by exogenous pathogenic factors, traumatic injuries or internal damage to the three passages, two channels and zang-fu organs, cause the dragon and fire channels in the lumbar region to be blocked, resulting in dysfunction or the inadequate nourishment of the related segments of the two channels. Consequently, qi stagnation and blood stasis occur in the lower back, leading to lumbago. In a word, in most cases, the mechanism of lumbago is qi stagnation and blood stasis, which is often accompanied by debilitation of qi and blood.

3. 诊察要点

1.3　Essentials for diagnosis

（1）诊断依据。

(1) Diagnosis criteria.

① 壮医诊断依据。参照《中国壮医外科学》（国家中医药管理局民族医药文献整理丛书，北京大学出版社、北京大学医学出版社，2018 年）。

① Diagnosis criteria in ZM: Diagnosis is established based on *Surgery of China's Zhuang Medicine*, one book in the ethnic medicine document series of State Administration of Traditional Chinese Medicine, published by Peking University Press, Peking University Medical Press in 2018.

主症：腰痛或伴有下肢放射性疼痛，呈阵发或持续性。

Main symptoms: Intermittent or persistent pain in the lower back, which may radiate along the lower limbs.

兼症：甚者可见转侧不利，仰俯不便，肌肉萎缩等。

Concurrent symptoms: Difficulty turning the body to the side and bending it forward and backward, muscle atrophy.

目诊：可见勒答白睛上 12 点脊柱反应区脉络迂曲，增多，散乱或集中，颜色浅或深，或白睛上有瘀斑。

Eye examination: More blood vessels on the reflex area (at the 12 o'clock position) to the spine on the white of the eyes are visible, curved, scattered or twisted, and light- or dark-colored. There may be ecchymosis on the white of the eyes.

甲诊：可见甲色淡或鲜红色，按压甲尖放开后恢复原色慢或快。

Nail examination: The nails are pale or bright red. When a fingernail stops being pressed, the color of the fingernail will return slowly or quickly.

舌脉象：舌质淡或暗，苔薄或腻，舌下脉络迂曲；脉沉细或涩。

Tongue and pulse examination: Pale or dark tongue with thin or greasy coating, curved blood vessels on the lower surface of the tongue, deep thready or choppy pulse.

② 中医诊断依据。参照全国中医药行业高等教育"十三五"规划教材《中医内科学》第十版。腰痛又称腰脊痛，是以腰脊或脊旁部位疼痛为主要表现的病证。

② Diagnosis criteria in TCM: Diagnosis is established based on *Internal Science of Traditional Chinese Medicine (10th Edition)*, a textbook in the series for the 13th Five-Year Plan of higher education for the national Chinese medicine industry. Lumbago, also known as lower back pain, is manifested by pain in the lumbar spine or paraspinal areas.

③ 西医诊断依据。参照《实用诊断学》（潘祥林，王鸿利主编，人民卫生出版社，2014 年）。腰椎间盘突出症以腰痛和坐骨神经痛为主要表现，有时疼痛剧烈，咳嗽、喷嚏时疼痛加重，卧床休息可缓解，会出现下肢麻木、有冷感或间歇性跛行等症状。青壮年多见，以 L4-S1 易发，患者常有搬重物史或扭伤史，可突发或缓慢发病。

③ Diagnosis criteria in WM: Diagnosis is established based on *Practice of Diagnostics*, edited by Pan Xianglin and Wang Hongli, and published by the People's Medical Publishing House in 2014. Lumbar disc herniation is mainly manifested by low back pain and sciatica, which become worse sometimes. The pain can be aggravated by coughing or sneezing, but relieved by bed rest. It may be accompanied by lower extremity numbness, a sensation of cold or intermittent claudication. It typically occurs at the L4-S1 in young adults, many of whom often carry heavy objects or have a history of sprains. The pain can come on suddenly or develop slowly.

（2）病证鉴别。

(2) Syndrome differentiation.

① 腰痛与背痛。腰痛是指腰背及其两侧部位的疼痛，背痛为背膂以上部位疼痛。

① Lumbago is characterized by pain in the lumbar region while back pain occurs in the posterior part of the upper trunk.

② 腰痛与尻痛。腰痛是指腰背及其两侧部位的疼痛，尻痛是尻骶部位的

疼痛。

② Lumbago is characterized by pain in the lumbar region while lumbosacral pain occurs in the sacral region.

③ 腰痛与胯痛。腰痛是指腰背及其两侧部位的疼痛，胯痛是指尻尾以下及两侧胯部的疼痛。

③ Lumbago is characterized by pain in the lumbar region while hip pain refers to pain below the rump tail and on both sides of the crotch.

4. 辨证论治

1.4 Syndrome differentiation and treatment

（1）治疗原则。祛湿毒，除瘀毒，通调三道两路。

(1) Treatment principles. Remove dampness toxin and blood stasis, and regulate the three passages and two channels.

（2）证治分类。

(2) Classification of syndrome identification and treatment.

① 取穴原则。

① Principles of acupoints selection.

三道两路配穴：三道两路配穴是指谷道、水道、气道、龙路、火路的穴位互相配合应用的方法。三道两路中任一道路发生病变时，除取本道路的穴位外，还可配伍其他道路的穴位。例如谷道不通畅而出现胃痛等谷道疾病时，除取谷道的脐内环穴（脾胃），还可取两路的脐内环穴（心），或配两路的体穴内关。

Passage-channel point combination: Points in the grain, water and qi passages, and in the dragon and fire channels are coordinated with each other. When there are pathological changes in any of the passages or channels, points in the diseased passage or channel can be coordinated with corresponding points on other ones. For example, if stomachache caused by the blockage of the grain passage occurs, the points corresponding to the spleen and stomach on the umbilical inner ring can be coordinated with the one corresponding to the heart on the umbilical inner ring or Neiguan (PC 6).

三部配穴：三部配穴是指脐天部、人部、地部的穴位，或人体天部、人部、地部的穴位互相配合应用的配穴法，可以是某二部配伍，也可以是三部配伍。如胃痛属人部病变，可取位于人部的脐内环穴（脾胃），再配以位于脐天部的脐环穴（心），还可配位于人体地部的体穴足三里。

Three parts combination: The points in the upper, middle and lower parts of the umbilicus and those in the heaven, human and earth parts of the human body are coordinated with each other. For example, stomachache occurs in the human part, so the points corresponding to the spleen and stomach on the umbilical inner ring can be coordinated with the one corresponding to the heart on the umbilical ring and Zusanli (ST 36) in the earth part of the human body.

② 主穴。咪腰（肾）、巧坞（脑）、咪心头（心）、咪叠（肝）、咪背（胆）、咪隆（脾）、咪胴（胃）、咪虽（肠）等。

② Primary acupoints: Points on the umbilical rings are selected, including those respectively corresponding to the kidney, brain, heart, liver, gallbladder, spleen, stomach and intestines[*].

③ 辨证分型。

③ Syndrome differentiation.

阴证。起病缓慢，病程较长，反复发作，时重时轻，腰部疼痛，以隐痛、胀痛、空痛为主。舌质淡或暗，苔白或白腻，舌下脉络迂曲、色青紫，脉沉、弦、弱、涩等，目诊见勒答白睛上 12 点脊柱反应区脉络散乱迂曲，颜色较浅，或有瘀斑。甲诊可见甲色淡，按压甲尖放开后恢复原色慢。

Yin syndrome: Lumbago has a slow onset and long-term course. It may be manifested as a dull pain, a distending pain and an empty pain, which recurs and varies in intensity. The tongue is pale or dark with white or white and greasy coating. The bluish purple blood vessels on the lower surface of the tongue are curved. The pulse is deep, thready, weak and/or choppy. The eye examination shows the blood vessels on the reflex area (at the 12 o'clock position) to the spine on the white of the eyes are curved, disordered and light-colored, or with ecchymosis. The nail examination shows the nails are pale and when a fingernail stops being pressed, the

---

[*] The word "kidney" is pronounced "Miyao" in the Zhuang language, "brain" is pronounced "Qiaowu", "heart" is pronounced "Mixintou", "liver" is pronounced "Midie", "gallbladder" is pronounced "Mibei", "spleen" is pronounced "Milong", "stomach" is pronounced "Midong" and "intestines" is pronounced "Misui".

color of the fingernail will return slowly.

若为肾虚型，则主症：病程较长，反复发作，以腰部隐痛为主，伴腰膝酸软或无力等。

Kidney deficiency type. Main symptoms: Long-term course, repeated attacks, a dull pain, soreness or weakness in the lumbar region and knees.

治疗原则：调水道，通两路。

Treatment principles: Regulate the water passage and unblock the two channels.

取穴：咪腰（肾）、咪心头（心）、巧坞（脑）、咪钵（肺）等。

Acupoints selection: Points on the umbilical rings, respectively corresponding to the kidney, heart, brain and lung.

若为瘀毒型，则主症：病程较长，反复发作，腰痛如刺，痛有定处。

Blood stasis type. Main symptoms: Long-term course, recurrence, a stabbing and fixed pain in the lumbar region.

治疗原则：祛瘀毒，通两路。

Treatment principles: Remove blood stasis and unblock the two channels.

取穴：咪腰（肾）、咪心头（心）、咪叠（肝）等。

Acupoints selection: Points on the umbilical ring, respectively corresponding to the kidney, heart and liver.

阳证：起病较急，病程短，腰部疼痛，疼痛较剧烈，以刺痛、跳痛、绞痛为主。舌质红或暗紫，苔白腻或黄腻，舌下脉络迁曲、色青黑，脉数、洪大、滑等。目诊勒答白睛上12点脊柱反应区脉络增多、增粗，色暗红或鲜红，靠近瞳孔。甲诊见甲色鲜红，按压甲尖放开后恢复原色快。

Yang syndrome: Lumbago has a sudden onset and short-term course. It is characterized by intense pain which may be manifested as a intense stabbing pain, a throbbing pain and a colicky pain. The tongue is red or dark purple with white, greasy or yellow, greasy coating. The blood vessels on the lower surface of the tongue are black and curved. The pulse is rapid, surging, large and/or slippery. The eye examination shows that more blood vessels on the reflex area (at the 12 o'clock position) to the spine on the white of the eyes are visible, enlarged, dark or bright red, and close to the pupils. The nail examination shows the nails are bright red and when a fingernail stops being pressed, the color of the fingernail will return quickly.

此为湿热型。主症：病程短，腰部疼痛，疼痛较剧烈，重着而热，活动后或可减轻，伴身体困重、小便短赤等。

Dampness-heat type. Main symptoms: Short-term course, intense lumbago, heavy and heat sensations in the lower back which may be relieved after exertion, heavy sensation in the body, and scanty, yellow urine.

治疗原则：祛湿毒，通两路。

Treatment principles: Remove dampness and unblock the two channels.

取穴：咪腰（肾）、咪隆（脾）、咪胴（胃）、咪虽（肠）等。

Acupoints selection: Points on the umbilical rings, respectively corresponding to the kidney, spleen, stomach and intestines.

5. 预防调护

1.5 Prevention and care

（1）生活起居：嘱患者睡软硬适度的硬板床，避风寒。

(1) Daily life: Advise patients to sleep on a medium firm mattress and avoid wind and cold.

（2）饮食调理：清淡饮食。

(2) Dietary adjustments: Have a diet low in fat and salt.

（3）情志调摄：保持心情舒畅。

(3) Emotional adjustments: Stay in a good mood.

（4）运动康复：愈后 3 个月至半年内，应避免重体力劳动、剧烈体育运动和日常生活中弯腰搬提重物，坚持腰背肌锻炼和逐步进行较轻柔的、有规律的体育锻炼，如做三气养生操、做广播操、打太极拳、慢跑等。

(4) Sports rehabilitation: Avoid strenuous physical exertion and intense sports within three months to half a year after recovery. Do not lift a heavy object with forward bend. Keep strengthening the lumbar and back muscles, and work out regularly and gently, for example, doing Three Qi Health Exercises, radio calisthenics, Tai Chi and jogging.

6. 医案选读

1.6   Selected case readings

【病案一】

［Case 1］

莫某，女，56 岁，2020 年 7 月 3 日初诊。

Patient: Mo, a 56-year-old woman, her first visit was on July 3, 2020.

现病史：腰痛反复发作 5 年余，加重 3 天入院。5 年前抬举重物后出现腰痛，以腰酸痛为主，虽反复治疗，但症状仍有反复，伴有睡眠不好，每晚仅睡 4 ～ 5 小时，腰 4 ～ 5 右侧疼痛明显，舌质淡，苔薄白，脉沉细。

History of present illness: Lumbago has repeatedly attacked in the past five years. It became worse three days ago so she was admitted to the hospital. Five years ago, lumbago which was characterized by an aching pain occurred due to heavy object lifting. Every time the lower back pain occurred, she had treatment, but it recurred sooner or later. She could only have 4~5 hours of sleep every night due to obvious pain on the right side of L4 to L5.

Her tongue is pale with white, thin coating. Her pulse is deep and thready.

壮医诊断：核尹（肾虚型）。中医诊断：腰痛。西医诊断：腰椎间盘突出症。

Diagnosis in ZM:"Heyin" characterized by kidney deficiency.

Diagnosis in TCM: Lumbago.

Diagnosis in WM: Lumbar disc herniation.

治疗原则：调水道，通两路。

Treatment principles: Regulate the water passage and unblock the two channels.

取穴：脐内环穴（心、肾、脑、肺）、髀关、阿是穴、膝弯处各穴如委中、腰龙脊等。

Acupoints selection: Points on the umbilical inner ring, respectively corresponding to the heart, kidney, brain and lung, Biguan (ST 31), Ashi points on the affected area, points on the area of the popliteal crease such as Weizhong (BL 40) and points on the spine in the lumbar region.

手法：呼吸吐纳补法，补 4 次。

Acupuncture method: Reinforcing method by respiration, which is used for 4 times.

二诊（2020 年 7 月 5 日）：腰痛症状明显好转，继续针灸 1 次，取穴及手法同上。

Second visit (on July 5, 2020): The pain had been relieved greatly. The acupuncture was performed on the same points with the same acupuncture method.

三诊（2020 年 7 月 8 日）：腰痛基本消失，但睡眠改善不明显，加灸神门、内关，艾灸照海。

Third visit (on July 8, 2020): The pain had almost disappeared, but her sleep quality was still poor, so Shenmen (HT 7) and Neiguan (PC 6) were added for acupuncture and Zhaohai (KI 6) for moxibustion.

四诊（2020 年 7 月 10 日）：睡眠症状进一步改善。

Fourth visit (on July 10, 2020): Sleep quality had been improved.

继续治疗 3 次，每 2 天治疗 1 次，巩固疗效。经过治疗后，腰痛未见复发，睡眠正常，随访 3 月，疗效巩固。

Accordingly, the patient was treated onwards to consolidate the efficacy, one time every two days, three times in total. After the treatment, the pain did not recur and her sleep was normal. The curative effect was maintained in the 3-month follow-up.

【病案二】

［Case 2］

韦某，男，33 岁，2021 年 1 月 9 日初诊。

Patient: Wei, a 33-year-old man, his first visit was on January 9, 2021.

现病史：患者近 10 年来腰痛反复发作，以刺痛为主，夜间明显，疼痛向右下肢放射痛，否认其他疾病史，纳寐可，二便调。

History of present illness: The patient's lumbago has recurred in the past ten years. It was manifested by a stabbing pain which became more obvious at night and radiated to his right lower limb. He reported no history of other diseases, good appetite, restful sleep, normal urination frequency and regular bowel movements.

壮医诊断：核尹（瘀毒型）。中医诊断：腰痛。西医诊断：腰椎间盘突出症。

Diagnosis in ZM: "Heyin" characterized by blood stasis.

Diagnosis in TCM: Lumbago.

Diagnosis in WM: Lumbar disc herniation.

治疗原则：祛瘀毒，通两路。

Treatment principles: Remove blood stasis and unblock the two channels.

取穴：脐内环穴（心、肾、肝）、夹脊等。

Acupoints selection: Points on the umbilical inner ring, respectively corresponding to the heart, kidney and liver, and Jiaji (EX-B 2).

手法：针脐内环穴时向外斜刺，采用平补平泻手法。

Acupuncture method: Neutral reinforcing-reducing method with oblique insertion outwards for the points on the umbilical inner ring.

二诊（2021 年 1 月 12 日）：腰痛略减，继续针灸 1 次，取穴及手法同上。

Second visit (on January 12, 2021): The pain had been relieved slightly. The acupuncture was performed on the same points with the same acupuncture method once.

三诊（2021 年 1 月 15 日）：腰痛明显减轻。继续针灸 1 次，取穴及手法同上。

Third visit (on January 15, 2021): The pain had been relieved greatly. The acupuncture was performed on the same points with the same acupuncture method once.

四诊（2021 年 1 月 18 日）：腰痛基本消失，继续针灸 1 次，以巩固疗效。

Fourth visit (on January 18, 2021): The pain almost disappeared. The acupuncture was performed on the same points with the same acupuncture method to consolidate the efficacy once.

（二）活邀尹（项痹病）

2　Nape impediment ("Huoyaoyin" in ZM)

1. 疾病概述

2.1　General description

活邀尹指各种原因导致颈部肌筋失衡，筋结形成，两路不通，进而产生颈部疼痛，活动受限，头晕头痛等症状的一种病证。相当于中医的项痹病、西医的颈椎病。

"Huoyaoyin", also known as nape impediment in TCM and cervical spondylosis in WM, is manifested by pain in the neck, reduced range of motion of the neck, dizziness and headache. The symptoms occur when the two channels are blocked. The blockage is caused by musculotendinous nodulation due to an imbalance between muscles and tendons in the neck.

2. 病因病机

2.2　Cause and mechanism of disease

活邀尹发病的主要病因是本虚、气血不足。在三道两路不通畅、脏腑功能失调、久病体弱的基础上，经脉失去濡养，可致肢体筋膜弛缓；外感毒邪，跌仆损伤，痰湿凝阻，内伤三道两路、枢纽脏腑，使龙路和火路不通畅，阻滞于项部，局部龙路、火路功能失调或失养，气血瘀滞于颈椎而发为本病。病机多见气血瘀滞，常兼有气血偏衰。

Nape impediment occurs mainly due to weak constitution and the deficiency of qi and blood. Specifically, the blockage of the three passages and two channels, dysfunction of zang-fu organs and weak constitution due to long-term illness lead to nutrition loss of the meridians, resulting that the limb muscles and tendons sag. If the saggy muscles and tendons contract exogenous pathogenic factors or get injured due to fall, the dragon and fire channels will be blocked. The blockage of these two channels can also result from phlegm-dampness obstruction and internal damage to the three passages, two channels and zang-fu organs. Consequently, the flow of qi and blood will be obstructed. When stagnation occurs at the neck, these two channels in this segment will malfunction or lose nutrition, resulting in nape impediment. In a word, in most cases, the mechanism of this disease is qi stagnation and blood stasis, which is often accompanied by the debilitation of qi and blood.

3. 诊察要点

2.3　Essentials for diagnosis

（1）诊断依据。

(1) Diagnosis criteria.

① 壮医诊断依据。参照《中国壮医外科学》（国家中医药管理局民族医药文献整理丛书，北京大学出版社、北京大学医学出版社，2018 年）。

① Diagnosis criteria in ZM: Diagnosis is established based on *Surgery of*

China's Zhuang Medicine, one book in the ethnic medicine document series of State Administration of Traditional Chinese Medicine, published by Peking University Press, Peking University Medical Press in 2018.

主症：颈部或伴有上肢放射性疼痛，呈阵发或持续性。

Main symptoms: Intermittent or persistent pain in the neck, which may radiate along the upper limbs.

兼症：颈部肌肉僵硬，活动受限，头痛头晕等。

Concurrent symptoms: Neck muscle rigidity with reduced range of motion, headache and dizziness.

目诊：可见勒答白睛上 12 点脊柱反应区脉络迂曲，增多，散乱或集中，颜色浅或深，或白睛上有瘀斑。

Eye examination: More blood vessels on the reflex area (at the 12 o'clock position) to the spine on the white of the eyes are visible, curved, scattered or twisted, and light- or dark-colored. There may be ecchymosis on the white of the eyes.

甲诊：可见甲色淡或鲜红，按压甲尖放开后恢复原色慢或快。

Nail examination: The nails are pale or bright red. When a fingernail stops being pressed, the color of the fingernail will return slowly or quickly.

舌脉象：舌淡红或暗红，苔薄或腻；脉沉细或涩。

Tongue and pulse examination: Reddish or dark red tongue with thin or greasy coating, deep and thready or choppy pulse.

② 中医诊断依据。参照全国中医药行业高等教育"十三五"规划教材《针灸学》第十版。项痹病是以头颈部疼痛，活动不利，甚至肩背痛，或肢体一侧或两侧麻木疼痛，或头晕目眩，或下肢无力，步态不稳，甚至肌肉萎缩等为主要表现的病证。

② Diagnosis criteria in TCM: Diagnosis is established based on *The Acupuncture (10th Edition)*, a textbook in the series for the 13th Five-Year Plan of higher education for the national Chinese medicine industry. The manifestations of nape impediment include pain in the neck and head, reduced range of motion of the neck, even pain in the shoulder and back, or numb pain on one or both sides of the limbs, or dizziness with blurred vision, or rolling gait due to weakness in the lower limbs, and even muscle atrophy.

③ 西医诊断依据。参照《实用诊断学》（潘祥林，王鸿利主编，人民卫生出版社，2014 年）。颈椎病以颈痛伴上肢放射性疼痛为主要表现，疼痛可放射到肩部或枕顶部，并按神经根分布向下放射到前臂及手部，轻者为持续性酸痛，重者可如刀割样针刺痛，并可出现一定部位的运动和感觉障碍。

③ Diagnosis criteria in WM: Diagnosis is established based on *Practice of Diagnostics*, edited by Pan Xianglin and Wang Hongli and published by the People's Medical Publishing House in 2014. Cervical spondylosis is characterized by neck pain which usually radiates upwards to the shoulder or the top of the occiput and downwards to the forearm and hand along the nerve roots. Mild cervical spondylosis causes a persistent aching pain while severe one leads to a knife-like stabbing pain which may be accompanied by motor and sensory disorders in some parts.

（2）病证鉴别。

(2) Syndrome differentiation.

① 神经根型颈椎病与尺神经炎鉴别。尺神经炎患者多有肘部神经沟压痛，且可触及条索状变性的尺神经，无前臂麻木，可通过发病部位及肌电图进行鉴别。

① Check the place where the disease begins and use the electromyography to distinguish cervical radiculopathy from ulnar neuritis which is a condition where pain normally occurs when the cubital tunnel is pressed and stripe-shaped ulnar nerves can be felt, but without forearm numbness.

② 颈性眩晕与耳源性眩晕鉴别。耳源性眩晕有三大临床特点：发作性眩晕、耳鸣、感应性进行性耳聋。而颈性眩晕同头颈转动有关，耳鸣程度轻。

② Otogenic vertigo is a condition characterized by sudden episodes of dizziness, tinnitus and progressive sensorineural hearing loss. On the other hand, dizziness caused by vertebral artery cervical spondylosis is associated with head and neck rotation, with mild tinnitus.

③ 脊髓型颈椎病与脊髓肿瘤鉴别。脊髓肿瘤可同时出现感觉障碍和运动障碍，病情呈进行性加重，对非手术治疗无效，应用磁共振成像可鉴别。

③ Magnetic resonance imaging can be used to differentiate cervical spondylotic myelopathy from a spinal cord tumor which may lead to sensory changes and motor disturbances at the same time, grows over time and cannot be treated with a non-surgical approach.

④ 交感型颈椎病与神经官能症鉴别。神经官能症没有颈椎病的 X 射线改变，无神经根和脊髓压迫症状，应用药物治疗有一定效果。

④ Sympathetic cervical spondylosis is different from neurosis. An X-ray image of sympathetic cervical spondylosis shows changes in the spine with compression of nerve roots and the spinal cord. On the other hand, neurosis does not have such symptoms. Its symptoms can be relieved with drugs.

4. 辨证论治

2.4　Syndrome differentiation and treatment

（1）治疗原则。气郁型以调气、通两路为主；瘀毒型以祛瘀毒、通两路为主；湿热型以祛湿毒、通两路为主。

(1) Treatment principles. For qi-depression type, adjust qi to unblock the two channels; for blood stasis type, remove blood stasis to unblock the two channels; for dampness-heat type, remove dampness to unblock the two channels.

（2）症治分类。

(2) Classification of syndrome identification and treatment.

① 取穴原则。

① Principles of acupoints selection.

三道两路配穴：三道两路配穴指谷道、水道、气道、龙路、火路的穴位互相配合应用的方法。三道两路中任一道路发生病变时，除取本道路的穴位外，还可配伍其他道路的穴位。例如谷道不通畅而出现胃痛等谷道疾病时，除取谷道的脐内环穴（脾胃）外，还可取两路的脐内环穴（心），或配两路的体穴内关。

Passage-channel point combination: Points in the grain, water and qi passages, and in the dragon and fire channels are coordinated with each other. When there are pathological changes in any of passages or channels, points in the diseased passage or channel can be coordinated with corresponding points on other ones. For example, if stomachache caused by the blockage of the grain passage occurs, the points corresponding to the spleen and stomach on the umbilical inner ring can be coordinated with the one corresponding to the heart on the umbilical inner ring or Neiguan (PC 6).

三部配穴：三部配穴是指脐天部、人部、地部的穴位，或人体天部、人部、地部的穴位互相配合应用的配穴法，可以是某二部配伍，也可以是三部配伍。如胃痛属人部病变，可取位于人部的脐内环穴（脾胃），再配以位于脐天部的脐环穴（心），还可配位于人体地部的体穴足三里。

Three parts combination: The points in the upper, middle and lower parts of the umbilicus and those in the heaven, human and earth parts of the human body are coordinated with each other. For example, stomachache occurs in the human part, so the points corresponding to the spleen and stomach on the umbilical inner ring can be coordinated with the one corresponding to the heart on the umbilical ring and Zusanli (ST 36) in the earth part of the human body.

② 主穴。巧坞（脑）、咪心头（心）、咪叠（肝）、咪背（胆）、咪隆（脾）、咪胴（胃）、咪虽（肠）等。

② Primary acupoints: Points on the umbilical rings, respectively corresponding to the brain, heart, liver, gallbladder, spleen, stomach and intestines.

③ 辨证分型。

③ Syndrome differentiation.

阴证：起病缓慢，病程较长，反复发作，时重时轻，颈部疼痛，疼痛以隐痛、胀痛、空痛为主。舌质淡或暗，苔白或白腻，舌下脉络迂曲、色青紫，脉沉、弦、弱、涩等，目诊见勒答白睛上 12 点脊柱反应区脉络散乱迂曲，颜色较浅，或有瘀斑。甲诊可见甲色淡，按压甲尖放开后恢复原色慢。

Yin syndrome: Cervical spondylosis has a slow onset and a long-term course. It is characterized by neck pain which recurs and varies in intensity. The pain may be manifested as a dull pain, a distending pain or an empty pain. The tongue is pale or dark with white or white and greasy coating. The blood vessels on the lower surface of the tongue are bluish purple and curved. The pulse is deep, thready, weak and/or choppy. The eye examination shows the blood vessels on the reflex area (at the 12 o'clock position) to the spine on the white of the eyes are curved and scattered, pale, or with ecchymosis. The nail examination shows the nails are pale and when a fingernail stops being pressed, the color of the fingernail will return slowly.

若为气郁型，则主症：颈部疼痛以胀痛、隐痛、空痛为主。

Qi-depression type. Main symptoms: Distending, dull or empty pain in the neck.

治疗原则：调气，通两路。

Treatment principles: Adjust qi to unblock the two channels.

取穴：巧坞（脑）、咪心头（心）、咪叠（肝）、咪背（胆）等。

Acupoints selection: Points on the umbilical rings, respectively corresponding to the brain, heart, liver and gallbladder.

若为瘀毒型，则主症：颈部疼痛如刺，痛有定处，痛处拒按。

Blood-stasis type. Main symptoms: Stabbing and fixed pain in the neck, resistance to pressure at the tender area.

治疗原则：祛瘀毒，通两路。

Treatment principles: Remove blood stasis to unblock the two channels.

取穴：巧坞（脑）、咪心头（心）、咪叠（肝）、咪隆（脾）、咪胴（胃）等。

Acupoints selection: Points on the umbilical rings, respectively corresponding to the brain, heart, liver, spleen and stomach.

阳证：起病较急，病程短，颈部疼痛，疼痛较剧烈，以刺痛、跳痛、绞痛为主。舌质红或暗紫，苔白腻或黄腻，舌下脉络迂曲、色青黑，脉数、洪大、滑等。目诊勒答白睛上 12 点脊柱反应区脉络增多、增粗，色暗红或鲜红，靠近瞳孔。甲诊见甲色鲜红，按压甲尖放开后恢复原色快。

Yang syndrome: Cervical spondylosis has a sudden onset and short-term course. It is characterized by an intense neck pain which may be manifested as a stabbing pain, a throbbing pain or a colicky pain. The tongue is red or dark purple with white greasy or yellow greasy coating. The blood vessels on the lower surface of the tongue are curved and bluish black. The pulse is rapid, surging, large and/or slippery. The eye examination shows that more blood vessels on the reflex area (at the 12 o'clock position) to the spine on the white of the eyes are visible, enlarged, dark or bright red, close to the pupils. The nail examination shows the nails are bright red and when a fingernail stops being pressed, the color of the fingernail will return quickly.

此为湿热型。主症：颈部疼痛明显，重着而热，暑湿阴雨天气加重，活动后或可减轻。

Dampness-heat type. Main symptoms: Obvious neck pain, heavy and heat sensations which are aggravated by summer-heat dampness and rainy weather, but may be relieved by exertion.

治疗原则：祛湿毒，通两路。

Treatment principles: Remove dampness to unblock the two channels.

取穴：巧坞（脑）、咪心头（心）、咪叠（肝）、咪隆（脾）、咪胴（胃）、咪虽（肠）等。

Acupoints selection: Points on the umbilical rings, respectively corresponding to the brain, heart, liver, spleen, stomach and intestines.

5. 预防调护

2.5　Prevention and care

（1）生活起居：避风寒，注意休息。

(1) Daily life: Avoid wind and cold, and have a good rest.

（2）饮食调理：清淡饮食。

(2) Dietary adjustments: Have a diet low in fat and salt.

（3）情志调摄：保持心情舒畅。

(3) Emotional adjustments: Stay in a good mood.

（4）运动康复：愈后 3 个月至半年内，应避免重体力劳动、剧烈体育运动和日常生活中长时间低头伏案工作，坚持进行颈部肌肉锻炼和做三气养生操。

(4) Sports rehabilitation: Avoid strenuous physical exertion, intense sports within three months to half a year after recovery; do not work with their heads down for a long time; and keep strengthening the neck muscles and work out regularly, for example, doing Three Qi Health Exercises.

6. 医案选读

2.6　Selected case readings

【病案一】

［Case 1］

苏某，2020 年 2 月 25 日初诊。

Patient: Su, the first visit was on February 25, 2020.

现病史：颈肩部疼痛 2 个月。自诉 2 个月前出现颈肩部疼痛，刺痛明显，右手拇指、食指麻木不适，无乏力，偶有头晕，无恶心呕吐等。

History of present illness: The patient reported an obvious stabbing pain that occurred in the neck and shoulders 2 months ago, acoompanied by numbness in the thumb and index finger of the right hand, absence of lassitude, occasional dizziness, and no nausea or vomiting.

壮医诊断：活邀尹（瘀毒型）。中医诊断：项痹病。西医诊断：颈椎病。

Diagnosis in ZM: "Huoyaoyin" characterized by blood stasis.

Diagnosis in TCM: Nape impediment.

Diagnosis in WM: Cervical spondylosis.

治疗原则：祛瘀毒，通两路。

Treatment principles: Remove blood stasis and unblock the two channels.

取穴：脐内环穴（脑、心、肝、脾、胃）、扁担穴、肩胛环穴、项棱穴、大椎、阿是穴等。

Acupoints selection: Points on the umbilical inner ring, respectively corresponding to the brain, heart, liver, spleen and stomach, Biandan*, points around the scapula, points on the ridge of the neck**, Dazhui (GV 14), Ashi points in the affected area.

手法：针脐内环穴，向外斜刺，采用平补平泻手法（图 17）。

Acupuncture method: Neutral reinforcing-reducing method with oblique insertion outwards for the points on the umbilical inner ring (Fig. 17).

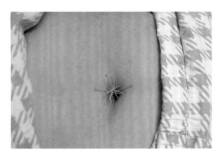

图 17　针脐内环穴

Fig. 17　Acupuncture at the points on the umbilical inner ring

---

* An acupoint uniquely applied in ZM, is on the place of a shoulder, where a carrying pole is put when it is used by people to carry a load.

** Refers to Jiaji (EX-B 2) near the neck in ZM.

二诊（2020年2月26日）：患者颈部疼痛略减，继续针灸1次，取穴及手法同上。

Second visit (on February 26, 2020): The neck pain had been relieved slightly. The acupuncture was performed on the same points with the same acupuncture method once.

三诊（2020年2月27日）：患者颈部疼痛明显减轻。继续针灸1次，取穴及手法同上。

Third visit (on February 27, 2020): The neck pain had been relieved greatly. The acupuncture was performed on the same points with the same acupuncture method once.

四诊（2020年2月29日）：患者颈部疼痛基本消失，继续针灸1次以巩固疗效。

Fourth visit (on February 29, 2020): The neck pain almost disappeared. The acupuncture was performed on the same points with the same acupuncture method to consolidate the efficacy once.

【病案二】

［Case 2］

李某，2020年3月2日初诊。

Patient: Li, the first visit was on March 2, 2020.

现病史：患者述5天前无明显诱因下出现颈部酸痛不适，伴有右上肢麻木。时有头晕，无头痛，无偏瘫。无咳嗽咳痰，无畏寒发热。无流行病学史。饮食睡眠欠佳，二便正常，舌淡，苔白，脉弦细。

History of present illness: The patient reported aching pain that occurred five days ago without any apparent reason, numbness in the right upper limb, occasional dizziness, no headache, no hemiplegia, no coughing, no sputum, no intolerance of cold and fever, no history of any infections, reduced appetite, restless sleep, normal urination frequency and regular bowel movements.

His tongue is pale with white coating. His pulse is thready and wiry.

壮医诊断：活邀尹（气郁型）。中医诊断：项痹病。西医诊断：颈椎病。

Diagnosis in ZM:"Huoyaoyin", characterized by qi-depression type.

Diagnosis in TCM: Nape impediment.

Diagnosis in WM: Cervical spondylosis.

治疗原则：调气，通两路。

Treatment principles: Adjust qi to unblock the two channels.

取穴：脐内环穴（脑、心、肝、胆）、扁担穴、肩胛环穴、项棱穴、大椎、阿是穴等。

Acupoints selection: Points on the umbilical inner ring, respectively corresponding to the brain, heart, liver and gallbladder, Biandan, points around the scapula, points on the ridge of the neck, Dazhui (GV 14), Ashi points in the affected area.

手法：针脐内环穴，向外斜刺，采用平补平泻手法（图 17）。

Acupuncture method: Neutral reinforcing-reducing method with oblique insertion outwards for the points on the umbilical inner ring (Fig. 17).

二诊（2020 年 4 月 7 日）：患者诉颈部疼痛明显缓解，继续针灸 1 次，取穴及手法同上。

Second visit (on April 7, 2020): The neck pain had been relieved greatly. The acupuncture was performed on the same points with the same acupuncture method once.

2020 年 4 月 30 日随访，患者诉针灸治疗后颈部疼痛基本消失。

Follow-up (on April 30, 2020): The patient reported that the pain in the nape almost disappeared.

（三）约经乱（月经不调）

3　Menstrual irregularities ("Yuejingluan" in ZM)

1. 疾病概述

3.1　General description

约经乱指月经周期、经量、经色等发生改变，并伴有其他症状。常见的有月经先期、月经后期、月经先后不定期等。月经先期指月经周期提前 7 天以上，甚至 10 余日一行。月经后期指月经周期延后 7 天以上，甚至 40 ～ 50 天一行。月经先后不定期指月经周期或提前或延后达 7 天以上。本病相当于中医的月经不调及西医的功能失调性子宫出血、生殖器炎症等引起的阴道异常出血。

Menstrual irregularities ("Yuejingluan" in ZM) is a general term for irregular menstruation and other menstrual complaints, such as abnormal duration, amount, and color of menstrual discharge. It includes polymenorrhea which refers to periods that come 7~10 days or more ahead of due time, oligomenorrhea which refers to periods that come 7 days or more, or even 40~50 days after due time, and irregular menstrual cycles which refer to periods that come with irregular cycles, more than 7 days earlier or later. It is also known as menstrual irregularities in TCM and abnormal vaginal bleeding caused by dysfunctional uterine bleeding, genital inflammation, etc.

2. 病因病机

3.2　Cause and mechanism of disease

约经乱发病的主要原因是本虚、脏腑功能失调、气血不足。脏腑功能失调，气血不足，三道两路不通畅，天、地、人三气不同步，"咪花肠"（胞宫）功能失调等均会导致经期异常。

Menstrual irregularities is caused by weak constitution, the dysfunction of zang-fu organs and the deficiency of qi and blood, which makes the three passages and two channels to be blocked. The blockage makes the heaven-qi, earth-qi and human-qi fail to synchronize with each other, resulting in the dysfunction of the uterus ("Mihuachang" in the Zhuang language). This ultimately leads to irregular menstruation.

3. 诊察要点

3.3　Essentials for diagnosis

（1）诊断依据。

(1) Diagnosis criteria.

参照《中医妇产科学》（第二版，刘敏如、谭万信主编，人民卫生出版社，2010 年）。

Diagnosis is established based on *Obstetrics and Gynecology of Traditional Chinese Medicine (2nd Edition)* edited by Liu Minru and Tan Wanxin, and published by the People's Medical Publishing House in 2010.

主症：月经先期、月经后期或月经先后不定期。

Main symptoms: Polymenorrhea, oligomenorrhea or irregular menstrual cycles.

兼症：经血量少或多、色鲜红或暗有块，少腹胀痛，乳胀胁痛，面色㿠白，神疲乏力，纳差，大便溏烂，腰膝酸痛等。

Concurrent symptoms: Light or heavy menstrual bleeding with bright red or dark red clots, lower abdominal distending pain, breast distension, hypochondriac pain, bright pale complexion, lassitude, reduced appetite, loose stool, aching pain in the lower back and knees.

目诊：可见勒答白睛上 6 点生殖器反应区脉络迂曲，增多，散乱或集中，颜色浅或深，或白睛上有瘀斑。

Eye examination: More blood vessels on the reflex area (at the 6 o'clock position) to the genitalia on the white of the eyes are visible, curved, scattered or twisted, and light-colored or dark-colored. There may be ecchymosis on the white of the eyes.

甲诊：可见甲色淡或鲜红，按压甲尖放开后恢复原色慢或快。

Nail examination: The nails are pale or bright red. When a fingernail stops being pressed, the color of the fingernail will return slowly or quickly.

舌脉象：舌淡红或暗红，苔薄或腻；脉沉细或涩。

Tongue and pulse examination: Reddish or dark red tongue with thin or greasy coating, and deep and thready, or choppy pulse.

① 月经先期。病史及临床表现：已婚育龄妇女常见有早期流产或习惯性流产及不孕史；基础体温（BBT）双相，但高温相评分（HPS）＜ 5，或 BBT 高温相短于 10 天，并持续 2 个周期以上；排卵后 6 天，两次血清孕酮量（P）＜ 10 ng/mL；经前期子宫内膜呈分泌期变化，但与正常月经周期的反应日期相差 2 天以上；黄体期卵巢二维超声检查显像见黄体表现而有临床症状；阴道涂片有时可见角化细胞指数偏高，细胞堆积，皱褶不佳。以上第二至第六项中有两项符合，结合临床，即可诊断。

① Polymenorrhea: Clinical manifestations and the medical history that married women of reproductive age have a history of early or recurrent pregnancy loss, or infertility.

The pattern of the basal body temperature (BBT) is biphasic, but high temperature phase score (HPS) is ＜ 5 or BBT high temperature phase lasts for less than 10 days in two consecutive cycles or more.

Six days after ovulation, the results of two tests show that the serum progesterone level is $<$ 10 ng/mL.

Before the period, the secretory change in the endometrium starts 2 days or earlier than that occurring under normal menstrual conditions.

In the luteal phase, ovarian B-scan ultrasonography shows the signs of a luteal phase defect.

Vaginal smears sometimes show a high keratinocyte index, and crowded and folded cells.

Polymenorrhea can be identified as long as two of the above items are included except the first one.

② 月经后期。

② Oligomenorrhea.

病史、临床表现。

Clinical manifestations and the medical history.

妇科检查：阴道窥器检查及盆腔内诊检查提示子宫大小正常或略小，余无明显阳性体征。

Gynecological examination: The vaginal speculum examination and pelvic examination show that the size of the uterus is normal or slightly small, without obvious positive signs.

辅助检查：妊娠试验多次阴性，二维超声检查子宫、附件有无发育不良或包块等病变，包括子宫大小、内膜厚度等；动态检测基础体温、阴道上皮脱落细胞、宫颈黏液形态以及生殖内分泌激素等以了解性腺轴功能，常常有卵泡发育延迟的情况存在。

Auxiliary examination: The results of several pregnancy tests are negative. B-scan ultrasonography checks the uterus and its appendages for lesions such as dysplasia and mass, as well as the uterine size and endometrial thickness. The dynamic testing is used to exam BBT, vaginal epithelial exfoliated cells, cervical mucus morphology, and reproductive endocrine hormones to understand the function of the gonadal axis. Follicle development is often found to be delayed.

③ 月经先后不定期。

③ Irregular menstrual cycles.

病史：可有不孕史或自然流产史。

The medical history: Have a history of infertility or spontaneous abortion.

妇科检查：内外生殖器官无器质性病变存在。

Gynecological examination: No organic lesions in internal and external reproductive organs.

辅助检查：内分泌激素测定，月经周期中不能形成黄体生成素（LH）高峰，卵巢不能排卵；或虽有排卵，但早期卵泡刺激素（FSH）相对不足，使卵泡发育延迟；或黄体期 LH 相对不足，黄体不健。基础体温测定为单相，或虽为双相，但低温相期过长或过短，或黄体期过短，高低温差小于 0.3 ℃。经潮 6 小时内子宫内膜活检，有排卵者，在延后周期可显示正常黄体分泌功能不足，在提前周期可显示黄体分泌功能不足；无排卵者则呈增生期改变。

Auxiliary examination: The hormone levels tests are conducted to show that luteinizing hormone (LH) secretion cannot surge to high levels around the midpoint of a cycle and thus ovulation cannot be triggered; that although ovulation occurs, follicle-stimulating hormone (FSH) is relatively insufficient in the early stage, which delays the development of follicles; or that LH deficiency during the luteal phase leads to corpus luteum insufficiency. The pattern of BBT is monophasic or biphasic. However, although it is biphasic, BBT low temperature phase lasts too long or too short, or the luteal phase is so short that the high-low temperature spread is less than 0.3 ℃. The results of an endometrial biopsy conducted within 6 hours after menstruation comes show that for those with ovulation, the progesterone secretion from their corpus luteum is deficient and for those without ovulation, their endometrium undergoes proliferative change.

（2）病证鉴别。

(2) Syndrome differentiation.

① 月经先期与经间期出血鉴别。月经先期患者，血量多少不定，出血持续时间多在 3 ～ 7 天内。经间期出血患者常表现为出血时间短，血量偏少。BBT 测定有助于诊断与鉴别。

① For polymenorrhea, although the blood volume varies, the bleeding duration is mostly within 3 to 7 days. On the other hand, for intermenstrual bleeding, the bleeding lasts short and the blood volume is low. BBT is an aid for diagnosis and differentiation.

② 月经后期与妊娠期出血鉴别。如既往月经周期及量、色、质均正常，本次月经延后一至数周又出现阴道流血，量、色、质均与以往不一样，或伴小腹疼痛但不同于以往经行腹痛特点，应注意与流产的各种临床类型如胎漏、胎动不安、堕胎、小产及宫外孕流产或破裂等妊娠有关病证相区别；若月经延后又伴有少量阴道出血和小腹疼痛，尤应注意与异位妊娠相区别。

② Bleeding during pregnancy is different from oligomenorrhea. For a patient, her previous menstrual cycles, and the amount, color and quality of menstrual discharge are normal, but vaginal bleeding occurs after this menstruation is delayed for one to several weeks, with the different blood amount, color and quality. She may also have abdominal pain which is different from that during menstruation. Accordingly, she may experience pregnancy-related disorders, including vaginal bleeding during pregnancy, threatened miscarriage, abortion, miscarriage and ectopic pregnancy. If the late period is accompanied by a small amount of vaginal bleeding and abdominal pain, it is essential to differentiate whether she experiences oligomenorrhea or ectopic pregnancy.

③ 月经先后不定期与崩漏鉴别。月经先后不定期为月经连续 3 个周期提前或延后 7 天以上，经期和经量基本正常。如伴经血暴下不止或淋漓持续难净，则属崩漏范畴。

③ Irregular menstrual cycles refer to periods that come with three irregular cycles in a row, more than 7 days earlier or later. On the other hand, massive or incessant extramenstral vaginal bleeding are the symptoms of metrorrhagia and metrostaxis.

4. 辨证论治

3.4　Syndrome differentiation and treatment

（1）治疗原则。气郁型以疏肝解郁、调气通经为主；脾肾虚型以补脾益肾、通调三道两路为主；气血虚型以平衡气血、通调三道两路为主；血寒型以温经散寒调经为主；阴虚型以平衡脏腑阴阳为主；血热型以清热解毒调经为主。

(1) Treatment principles. For qi-depression type, smooth the liver, relieve depression and adjust qi to unblock the two channels; for spleen-kidney deficiency type, tonify the spleen, replenish the kidney and regulate the three passages and two channels; for qi-blood deficiency type, harmonize qi with blood and regulate the three passages and two channels; for blood-cold type, warm the meridians/channels and dissipate cold to regulate menstruation; for yin-deficiency type, balance yin and yang of zang-fu organs; for blood-heat type, clear away heat, resolve toxins to regulate menstruation.

（2）症治分类。

(2) Classification of syndrome identification and treatment.

① 取穴原则。

① Principles of acupoints selection.

三道两路配穴：三道两路配穴指谷道、水道、气道、龙路、火路的穴位互相配合应用的方法。三道两路中任一道路发生病变时，除取本道路的穴位外，还可配伍其他道路的穴位。例如谷道不通畅而出现胃痛等谷道疾病时，除取谷道的脐内环穴（脾胃），还可取两路的脐内环穴（心），或配两路的体穴内关。

Passage-channel point combination: Points in the grain, water and qi passages, and in the dragon and fire channels are coordinated with each other. When there are pathological changes in any of passages or channels, the points in the diseased passage or channel can be coordinated with corresponding points on other ones. For example, if stomachache caused by the blockage of the grain passage occurs, the points corresponding to the spleen and stomach on the umbilical inner ring can be coordinated with the one corresponding to the heart on the umbilical inner ring or Neiguan (PC 6).

三部配穴：三部配穴是指脐天部、人部、地部的穴位，或人体天部、人部、地部的穴位互相配合应用的配穴法，可以是某二部配伍，也可以是三部配伍。如胃痛属人部病变，可取位于人部的脐内环穴（脾胃），再配以位于脐天部的脐环穴（心），还可配位于人体地部的体穴足三里。

Three parts combination: The points in the upper, middle and lower parts of the umbilicus and those in the heaven, human and earth parts of the human body are coordinated with each other. For example, stomachache occurs in the human part, so the point corresponding to the spleen and stomach on the umbilical inner ring can be coordinated with the one corresponding to the heart on the umbilical ring and Zusanli (ST 36) in the earth part of the human body.

② 主穴。咪腰（肾）、咪小肚（膀胱）、咪花肠（胞宫）、咪心头（心）、咪叠（肝）、咪背（胆）、咪隆（脾）、咪胴（胃）等。

② Primary acupoints: Points on the umbilical rings, respectively corresponding to the kidney, bladder, womb*, heart, liver, gallbladder, spleen and stomach.

③ 辨证分型。

③ Syndrome differentiation.

阴证：月经先期、月经后期或月经先后不定期，伴有经血量少或多，色淡或暗有块，少腹胀痛，乳胀胁痛，面色㿠白，神疲乏力，纳差，大便溏烂，腰膝酸痛等。目诊可见勒答白睛上 6 点生殖器反应区脉络迂曲，增多，散乱，颜色浅，或白睛上有瘀斑。甲诊可见甲色淡，按压甲尖放开后恢复原色慢。舌淡红或暗红，苔薄或腻，脉沉细或涩。

Yin syndrome: Polymenorrhea, oligomenorrhea and irregular menstrual cycles, light or heavy menstrual bleeding with bright red or dark red clots, lower abdominal distending pain, breast distension, hypochondriac pain, bright pale complexion, lassitude, reduced appetite, loose stool, aching pain in the lower back and knees, etc. The eye examination shows that more blood vessels on the reflex area (at the 6 o'clock position) to the genitalia on the white of the eyes are visible, curved, scattered, and light-colored or dark-colored, or with ecchymosis on the white of the eyes. The nail examination shows the nails are pale or bright red, and when a fingernail stops being pressed, the color of the fingernail will return slowly. The tongue is reddish or dark red with thin or greasy coating. The pulse is deep and thready, or choppy.

若为气郁型，则主症：月经先后不定期，量少色暗有块，排出不畅，伴有小腹胀痛，乳胀胁痛等。

---

* The word "bladder" is pronounced "Mixiaodu" in the Zhuang language and "womb" is pronounced "Mihuachang".

Qi-depression type. Main symptoms: Irregular menstrual cycles, light menstrual bleeding with dark red clots and poor flow, lower abdominal distending pain, breast distension and hypochondriac pain.

治疗原则：调气，通三道两路。

Treatment principles: Adjust qi to unblock the three passages and two channels.

取穴：脐内环穴（胞宫、肾、肝、胆）、太冲、曲泉、妇科穴等。

Acupoints selection: Points on the umbilical inner ring, respectively corresponding to the womb, kidney, liver and gallbladder, Taichong (LR 3), Ququan (LR 8) and points usually used for gynecological diseases.

若为脾肾虚型，则主症：月经先期、月经后期或月经先后不定期，伴有纳差，大便溏烂，腰膝酸痛等。

Spleen-kidney deficiency type. Main symptoms: Polymenorrhea, oligomenorrhea, irregular menstrual cycles, reduced appetite, loose stool, aching pain in the lower back and knees.

治疗原则：调水道，补益脾肾。

Treatment principles: Regulate the water passage and tonify the spleen and kidney.

取穴：脐内环穴（胞宫、肾、脾、胃）、三阴交、太溪、气海、关元等。

Acupoints selection: Points on the umbilical inner ring, respectively corresponding to the womb, kidney, spleen and stomach, Sanyinjiao (SP 6), Taixi (KI 3), Qihai (CV 6) and Guanyuan (CV 4).

气血虚型。主症：月经后期或月经先后不定期，月经量少，色淡，面色㿠白，神疲乏力，心悸气短，食欲不振，舌淡苔薄，脉细弱无力。

Qi-blood deficiency type. Main symptoms: Oligomenorrhea, irregular menstrual cycles, a small amount of pale red bloody discharge, bright pale complexion, lassitude, palpitation, shortness of breath, reduced appetite, pale tongue with thin coating, and thready, weak pulse.

治疗原则：调水道，补益气血。

Treatment principles: Regulate the water passage and tonify qi and blood.

取穴：脐内环穴（胞宫、肾、肝、脾、胃）、气海、关元、妇科穴等。

Acupoints selection: Points on the umbilical inner ring, respectively corresponding to the womb, kidney, liver, spleen and stomach, Qihai (CV 6), Guanyuan (CV 4) and points usually used for gynecological diseases.

若为血寒型，则主症：月经后期或月经先后不定期，量少色暗，有块，或色淡质稀，伴有小腹冷痛，喜温喜按，得热则减，或畏寒肢冷。

Blood-cold type. Main symptoms: Oligomenorrhea, irregular menstrual cycles, a small amount of dark red bloody discharge with clots, or watery pale red bloody discharge, lower abdominal cold pain which can be relieved by heat, has a preference for heat and pressure, or intolerance of cold and cold extremities.

治疗原则：调水道，祛寒毒。

Treatment principles: Regulate the water passage and remove cold.

取穴：脐内环穴（胞宫、肾、脾、胃）、三阴交、气海、关元、大敦等。

Acupoints selection: Points on the umbilical inner ring, respectively corresponding to the womb, kidney, spleen and stomach, Sanyinjiao (SP 6), Qihai (CV 6), Guanyuan (CV 4) and Dadun (LR 1).

若为阴虚型，则主症：月经先期，月经量不多甚至减少，色鲜红质稠，伴有面潮红，手足心热，盗汗，心烦失眠，口干。

Yin-deficiency type. Main symptoms: Polymenorrhea, a small or even less amount of thick bright red bloody discharge, flushed face, feverish sensation in the palms and soles, night sweats, vexation, insomnia and thirst.

治疗原则：调水道，平衡气血阴阳。

Treatment principles: Regulate the water passage and balance qi and blood, as well as yin and yang.

取穴：脐内环穴（胞宫、肾、脾、胃）、三阴交、气海、关元、妇科穴等。

Acupoints selection: Points on the umbilical inner ring, respectively corresponding to the womb, kidney, spleen and stomach, Sanyinjiao (SP 6), Qihai (CV 6), Guanyuan (CV 4) and points usually used for gynecological diseases.

阳证：月经先期，血色鲜红，量多，湿热内蕴，烦躁易怒，口渴。舌红，苔黄腻，脉滑数。目诊见勒答白睛上6点生殖器反应区脉络增粗曲张，边缘混浊，多而集中靠近瞳仁，色深。甲诊见甲色鲜红，按压甲尖放开后恢复原色快。

Yang syndrome: Polymenorrhea, a large amount of bright red bloody discharge, internal retention of dampness-heat, vexation, irritability, thirst, red tongue with yellow and greasy coating, slippery and rapid pulse. The eye examination shows that on the reflex area (at the 6 o'clock position) to the genitalia on the white of the eyes, the blood vessels with turbid edges are enlarged, curved and twisted, many of which are close to the pupils. The nail examination shows the nails are bright red and when a fingernail stops being pressed, the color of the fingernail will return quickly.

此为血热型。主症：月经先期，血色鲜红，量多，湿热内蕴，面赤，烦躁易怒，口渴。

Blood-heat type. Main symptoms: Polymenorrhea, a large amount of bright red bloody discharge, internal retention of dampness-heat, flushed face, vexation, irritability and thirst.

治疗原则：调水道，祛热毒。

Treatment principles: Regulate the water passage and clear away heat.

取穴：脐内环穴（胞宫、肾、脾、胃）、三阴交、妇科穴、太冲、丰隆等。

Acupoints selection: Points on the umbilical inner ring, respectively corresponding to the womb, kidney, spleen and stomach, Sanyinjiao (SP 6), Taichong (LR 3), Fenglong (ST 40) and points usually used for gynecological diseases.

5. 预防调护

3.5   Prevention and care

（1）生活起居。避风寒，注意休息。

(1) Daily life: Avoid wind and cold, and have a good rest.

（2）饮食调理：忌食辛辣刺激寒凉饮食。

(2) Dietary adjustments: Avoid spicy, stimulating and cold foods.

（3）情志调摄。保持心情舒畅。

(3) Emotional adjustments: Stay in a good mood.

（4）避免重体力劳动或剧烈运动。

(4) Avoid strenuous physical exertion or intense sports.

6. 医案选读

3.6　Selected case readings

【病案一】

［Case 1］

黄某，2021 年 4 月 27 日初诊。

Patient: Huang, her first visit was on April 27, 2021.

现病史：自述 10 个月前停避孕药后出现月经后期，月经期 5 ～ 7 天，色红，量可，无痛经，颈背酸累，无头痛头晕，无胸闷心慌，平素脾气急，纳可，寐欠佳，小便调，大便溏。

History of present illness: The patient reported late periods after she stopped taking contraceptives ten months ago, 5~7 days of menstruation with a normal amount of red bloody discharge, absence of abdominal menstrual pain, soreness and weakness in the neck and back, no headache, no dizziness, no chest stuffiness, no palpitation, quick temper, good appetite, restless sleep, normal urination frequency and loose stool.

壮医诊断：约经乱（脾肾虚型）。中医诊断：月经不调。西医诊断：功能失调性子宫出血。

Diagnosis in ZM: "Yuejingluan" characterized by spleen-kidney deficiency.

Diagnosis in TCM: Menstrual irregularities.

Diagnosis in WM: Dysfunctional uterine bleeding.

治疗原则：调水道，补益脾肾。

Treatment principles: Regulate the water passage and tonify the spleen and kidney.

取穴：脐内环穴（胞宫、肾、脾、胃）、三阴交、太溪、气海、关元等。

Acupoints selection: Points on the umbilical inner ring, respectively corresponding to the womb, kidney, spleen and stomach, Sanyinjiao (SP 6), Taixi (KI 3), Qihai (CV 6) and Guanyuan (CV 4).

手法：针脐内环穴，向外斜刺，采用补法（图 18）。

Acupuncture method: Reinforcing method with oblique insertion outwards for the points on the umbilical inner ring (Fig. 18).

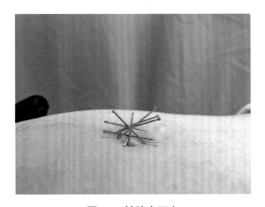

图 18　针脐内环穴

Fig. 18　Acupuncture at the points on the umbilical inner ring

二诊（2021 年 5 月 5 日）：患者诉未行经，继续针灸 1 次，取穴及手法同上。

Second visit (on May 5, 2021): The patient reported the period had not come yet. The acupuncture was performed on the same points with the same acupuncture method once.

三诊（2021 年 5 月 13 日）：患者诉未行经，继续针灸 1 次，取穴及手法同上。

Third visit (on May 13, 2021): The patient reported the period had not come yet. The acupuncture was performed on the same points with the same acupuncture method once.

【病案二】

［Case 2］

李某，2021 年 7 月 23 日初诊。

Patient: Li, her first visit was on July 23, 2021.

现病史：末次月经为 2021 年 7 月 7 日，淋漓不尽至今，色暗红，量少。平素怕冷，2 周前受寒出现咳嗽，有痰难咳出，大小便正常，舌质红，苔白腻，右寸尺沉细濡、关弦，左寸尺沉细、关濡。12 岁初潮。

History of present illness: The patient reported her last menstrual period (LMP) started on July 7 2021 but lasted until now. Her bloody discharge was dark red, with a small amount, and she had intolerance of cold. She experienced cough that occurred due to exogenous cold two weeks ago. Her sputum was hard to be brought up by cough. Her urination frequency was normal and bowel movements were regular. Her tongue is red with white, greasy coating. Her right Cun pulse is deep, thready and soggy, and right Guan pulse is wiry. Her left Cun pulse is deep, thready and left Guan pulse is soggy. She reported she got her first period when she was 12 years old.

壮医诊断：约经乱（血寒型）。中医诊断：月经不调。西医诊断：功能失调性子宫出血。

Diagnosis in ZM:"Yuejingluan", characterized by blood cold.

Diagnosis in TCM: Menstrual irregularities.

Diagnosis in WM: Dysfunctional uterine bleeding.

治疗原则：调水道，祛寒毒。

Treatment principles: Regulate the water passage and remove cold.

取穴：脐内环穴（胞宫、肾、脾、胃）、三阴交、气海、关元、大敦等。

Acupoints selection: Points on the umbilical inner ring, respectively corresponding to the womb, kidney, spleen and stomach, Sanyinjiao (SP 6), Qihai (CV 6), Guanyuan (CV 4) and Dadun (LR 1).

手法：针脐内环穴，向外斜刺，采用补法（图18）。

Acupuncture method: Reinforcing method with oblique insertion outwards for the points on the umbilical inner ring (see Fig. 18).

二诊（2021年7月27日）：患者诉月经淋漓不尽，量较前减少，继续针灸1次，取穴及手法同上。

Second visit (on July 27, 2021): The patient reported her period was still incessant but the amount of blood discharge had decreased. The acupuncture was performed on the same points with the same acupuncture method once.

三诊（2021年8月2日）：患者诉月经已停未行经，继续针灸1次，取穴及手法同上，以巩固疗效。

Third visit (on August 2, 2021): The patient reported her period had ended. The acupuncture was performed on the same points with the same acupuncture method to consolidate the efficacy once.

第四章　壮医药浴疗法
Chapter 4　Zhuang Medicine Medicated Bath Therapy

一、疗法概况
Ⅰ　Introduction

（一）发展历史
1　History of the Zhuang medicine medicated bath therapy

　　壮医药浴疗法一直流传于壮族民间，历史悠久，源远流长。在中华人民共和国成立前，壮族虽有壁画文字，但大多数人不甚理解，族内人民往往是通过语言进行交流，一些行之有效的药浴偏方、验方只能靠口头流传形成一定的习俗，较少见诸文字记载。考古资料证明，壮医药浴疗法远在石器时代壮族先民学会用火之时已有萌芽，是千百年来壮族人民赖以防病治病的有效手段和方法之一。农历五月初五靖西端午药市开市，自由市场摆满各种各样的中草药供人们购买，靖西的壮族人民至今还保留着在这天进行药浴的习俗，他们会自行上山采药或到药市采购，将草药合煮成一大锅药水，给全家淋浴或熏洗，以驱邪、健身、消灾保安、避疫气。此外，由于壮族是一个尚武民族，民风彪悍，壮族人民自幼练武强身，习武时也常用中草药泡洗全身，以消除疲惫，增强功力。直至今日，靖西、德保、田阳、百色一带习武的人仍习惯用草药泡洗或熏洗身体。

　　The Zhuang medicine (ZM) medicated bath therapy boasts a long history in treating the Zhuang people. Before the founding of the People's Republic of China, many special but irregular recipes and proven formulas for medicinal bath were merely handed down by word of mouth or by transforming into customs, because most of the Zhuang people were illiterate, although there was writing on murals. Archaeological evidence suggests that the ZM medicated bath therapy, an effective method used for thousands of years among the Zhuang people for disease prevention and treatment, dates back to the Stone Age when the Zhuang ancestors learned to use fire. The customs of having a herbal medicine fair and taking a medicinal bath on May 5th in lunar calendar are preserved all the time by the Zhuang people living in Jingxi, Guangxi. On that day, all family members take a medicinal bath or fumigation with decoction of Chinese herbs which are bought from the fairground or gathered in the mountain on their own. In this way, it is expected to remove evil spirits, strengthen the body, eliminate disasters and prevent epidemics. In addition, the Zhuang people advocate martial arts so many of them start to practice it in childhood. After practice, they often take a medicinal bath or fumigation to eliminate fatigue and enhance power. To date, people who practice martial arts in Jingxi, Debao, Tianyang and Bose still have such a habit.

《素问·异法方宜论》曾谓，南方乃天长地养、阳盛阴衰之地也，云雾缭绕，雨露聚集，此处之人易正气虚，而生瘴、盛、风、湿之病。其所言南方者，是为地处岭南、瘴气郁蒸的壮族地区。此处为草木水泉茂密之地，集天地阴恶之气，可使人阳气常外泄，遂使人夏不胜邪，冬不闭藏，人居其间，长此以往，乃日遭草木之阴毒，元气不能常固也。遂壮族之人，春生草瘴，夏生梅瘴，秋生禾瘴，冬生茅瘴，人多生疾病，而壮医始也。

According to *Su Wen·Yi Fa Fang Yi Lun (On Methods of Treatment in Plain Questions)*, in the southern region, it is warm most of the year, often cloudy and foggy, and abundant in rain and dew, so it is suitable for all living things to grow, but the healthy qi in people living there tends to be insufficient, resulting in diseases caused by miasma, yin exuberance, wind and dampness. The southern region described in the ancient document now refers to the settlements of the Zhuang nationality in Lingnan area, which is shrouded by miasma. In such a place, vegetation and springs are lush, resulting in the exuberance of yin qi and pathogenic qi in nature, which makes yang qi in the body spread outward. Thus, the human body fails to resist the invasion of pathogenic qi in summer and store yang qi in winter. If people live in such environment for a long time, original qi cannot be constantly arrested within the body, leading to diseases caused by green grass miasma in spring, Huangmei miasma in summer, Xinhe miasma in autumn, and Huangmao miasma in winter[*]. Consequently, ZM emerged.

　　壮医药浴疗法以壮医药理论为指导。壮医药理论首先讲究"天人自然观"，主张阴阳为本的思想。壮族人民聚居于亚热带，他们在这与世隔绝的山林之中，昼夜更替之际，冬去春来时候，摸索出了阴阳互换的道理。因此壮医笃信阴阳变化之理，其药浴之道亦视阴阳为本，乃调和阴阳、使之合二为一、相化相融的养生之法。其次，壮医所说之气，乃人体之气，壮医判定一个人生死与否，皆凭一气存否。气在一呼一吸之间，此乃壮医以气为要、以气为治之理。秉天地阴阳之气而长，食五谷之气而生，赖天地之源而用，故壮医以"气道""食道""水道"为人命之三道，其药浴文化亦秉持此理，打通人体之三道，令气机协调，谷道畅通，水道不滞，方可长寿。最后，壮医以治毒解毒为重，因其地处毒物甚多的岭南地带，毒虫、毒草、毒兽、毒物无所不在，此乃天地造化使然也，而治毒解毒之方药技法亦多。

The ZM theories provide a basis to the application of the ZM medicated bath therapy. First, ZM is characterized by the theory of correspondence between nature and human as the most important theory, and the concept of yin and yang as the fundamental principle. In ancient times, the Zhuang people experienced the day/night cycle and the alteration of seasons while living in subtropical mountain forests. Gradually, they understood mutual actions of yin and yang, naturally making ZM adhere to the concept of yin-yang interaction. Accordingly, the ZM medicated bath therapy is applied to regulate yin and yang to make them harmonious, thereby preserving health of the human body. Second, in ZM, qi normally refers to qi within the body. Its existence indicates whether a person is alive or not. The human body grows by breathing yang qi and yin qi from nature, taking qi of food and drinking water, so in ZM, the qi, grain and water passages are regarded as the basic elements which support vital activities of the body. Based on these thoughts, priority is given to the regulation of qi in Zhuang medical practices. Accordingly, this therapy is applied to unblock the three passages to maintain smooth qi movement. Only when

---

[*] "Huangmei" refers to the Huangmei season characterized by annoying continuous rain and high humidity; "Xinhe" means new grains; and "Huangmao" means yellow grass.

the grain passage and water passage are unobstructed, can longevity be reached. Third, there are a variety of poisons, including poisonous insects, weeds, beasts and food, in Lingnan area where the Zhuang people live. Such natural environment forced ZM practitioners to create many formulas to remove toxins and pay much attention to detoxication during disease treatment.

根据壮医药理论，壮医药浴疗法虽为外治之法，亦以平衡阴阳、调气、驱除邪毒为治病之道。其药浴所用之草药，因地而取，根据患者、患部、患机而取不同之浴药，以浸泡、蒸煮及热疗之法，作用于患处，可舒筋活络，调和气血，亦调节天、地、人三气之平衡，以期可清热解毒，消肿止痛，强身健体，活血行气，温经散寒及疏通经脉，最终使全身气机畅通，阴阳调和，脏腑无邪，两路无阻，达到抵御疾病、强身健体、调养身心之效果。

From the perspective of ZM, the ZM medicated bath therapy can balance yin with yang, adjust qi and remove pathogenic toxins, although it is an external treatment method. For different medical conditions, and disease sites and mechanisms, different herbs gathered at local places are applied with the mode of medicated bath, steam bath or hyperthermia to the affected area to relax tendons, activate the collaterals, harmonize qi and blood and make the heaven-qi, earth-qi and human-qi synchronized. Thus, it is expected to clear away heat, remove toxins, eliminate swelling, relieve pain, strengthen the body, activate blood, move qi, warm and unblock the meridians and collaterals and dissipate cold. This results in smooth qi movement, balance between yin and yang, healthy zang-fu organs without pathogenic qi and two smooth channels. In a word, the therapy can be used to prevent diseases, strengthen the body, and recuperate the body and mind.

近年来，随着人民生活水平的不断提高，人们对传统医学尤其是民族医学的重视程度越来越高，对包括壮医药浴疗法等民族医学预防疾病的方法更加重视。作为壮医药特色疗法之一的壮医药浴疗法在壮族地区得到较快的发展，已成为广大民众保健、康复的重要手段之一。

In the past decades, the improvement in the living standards have enabled people to pay more attention to disease prevention and health care. As a result, traditional medicines which provide many treatment methods to prevent diseases are drawing more and more attention. As a distinctive ZM therapeutic technique, the ZM medicated bath therapy has been greatly promoted in the settlements of the Zhuang nationality to become an important method for disease prevention and health care.

（二）治疗机理

2　Treatment mechanism

1. 皮肤透皮吸收

2.1　Transdermal absorption

皮肤为人体最大的器官，除能保护体内组织和器官免受外界各种刺激外，还有排泄和透皮吸收等作用。药物作用于皮肤，可通过局部的皮肤黏膜、汗腺、毛囊、角质层、细胞及其间隙等将药物转运而吸收进入人体。药浴时温热的药物能加强水合作用和皮肤的通透性，加速皮肤对药物的吸收，通过血液循环将药物散布到组织、器官而引起整体药理效应。

As the largest organ of the body, the skin protects the body tissues and organs from various external stimuli and functions in excretion and absorption. By stimulating the skin, medicine enters the body through local mucous membranes, sweat glands, hair follicles, stratum corneum, and cells and their gaps. When the body is soaked in the hot bath, the skin is hydrated and the high water temperature increases its permeability, resulting in acceleration of medicine absorption by the skin. Then, the medicine goes with the blood circulation to tissues and organs to achieve health effects.

2. 药物直接作用

2.2　Direct effects

对于局部性疾病，壮医药浴疗法用药贴近病灶，药力集中，奏效尤捷。治疗时熏洗局部（患处），将药物作用于局部组织，使局部组织的药物浓度高于其他部位，直达病所而起到清热解毒、消肿止痒、拔毒祛腐等作用。

Medicine can take intensive and quick efficacy on the diseased site because the skin is soaked in the medicinal soup. Steaming and washing the affected area makes medicine concentration on it higher than that on other areas, and enables the medicine to directly act on the site to clear away heat, remove toxins, eliminate swelling, relieve itching and draw out toxins to remove putridity.

3. 局部刺激

2.3　Regional stimulation

药浴时通过药温使皮肤温度升高，且在使用具有刺激作用的药物时，使局部血管扩张，促进血液及淋巴循环，改善周围组织的营养，从而起到消炎退肿的作用。温热药物对局部的刺激有类似灸法的效应，具有温经通络、行气活血、祛湿散寒的效果。温热刺激能促进网状内皮系统的吞噬功能，促进新陈代谢。对于真菌、细菌感染性疾病，药物药浴能直接起到抑制与杀灭真菌、细菌的作用。再者，药物作用于局部而引起的神经反射作用能激发机体的自身调节作用，促进机体某些抗体的形成，从而提高机体的免疫功能。

In medicated bath, by raising the skin temperature with high water temperature and stimulating the skin with medicine, blood vessels in the local area dilate, the circulations of blood and lymph are accelerated, and nutrients in the surrounding tissues increase. This will eliminate inflammation and swelling. As with the curative effectiveness of moxibustion, such treatment method can warm and unblock the meridians and collaterals, move qi, activate blood, remove dampness and dissipate cold. Thermal stimulation can enhance the phagocytic function of the reticuloendothelial system, accelerate metabolism, and inhibit and kill fungal and bacteria to treat fungal and bacterial infections. In addition, the reflexes caused by medicine acting on the local area can stimulate the body's self-regulation and make some antibodies form, resulting in boosting the immune system.

药浴通过疏通三道两路气机驱毒外出，可用于治疗疾病，亦可作为一种保健养生的手段。

The medicated bath therapy can be used to move qi in the three passages and two channels to expel toxins, so it can be a treatment method and a means of health care.

（三）主要功效

3　Main efficacy

1. 祛邪解毒

3.1　To disperse pathogenic qi and remove toxins

从外因来说，疾病的发生主要是受到痧、瘴、蛊、毒、风、湿等有形或无形之邪毒的侵犯，故治疗上重视散邪，以祛毒为先。壮医药浴疗法可通过药物与热力刺激，使毒、邪随汗液、尿液排出。

In terms of external factors, a disease is caused by invasion of visible or invisible pathogenic toxins such as filth, miasma, parasite, poison, wind and dampness. Therefore, ZM practitioners pay much attention to dispersing pathogens and give priority to detoxification. In the ZM medicated bath therapy, medicine and heat stimulation have a synergistic effect to remove toxins and disperse pathogens by sweating and urination.

2. 调气

3.2　To adjust qi

气血在人体内始终处于流动通畅的状态，才能营养全身，古有"气血贵流不贵滞"的说法，因此，治疗时必须十分注意气血以流通为贵的特性。气属阳，血属阴，气为血之帅，气行则血行。气血运行于脏腑之中，是内脏器官进行生理活动的基础。内脏居于体内，其生理病理变化可反映于外。壮医药浴疗法通过调节、激发或通畅人体之气，使之正常运行，与天地之气保持同步。

As the old saying goes, "It is essential to move qi and blood". In other words, only when qi and blood move smoothly, can the whole body obtain nutrients. Therefore, in treatment, Zhuang practitioners should pay close attention to the circulations of qi and blood. Qi is yang in nature while blood is yin in nature. Qi is the commander of blood, so when qi moves, blood circulates. Running through zang-fu organs, qi and blood are the dynamic forces of their physiological functions. Although zang-fu organs are within the body, their pathological changes can be manifested externally. The ZM medicated bath therapy can be used to adjust, stimulate or move qi to synchronize the human-qi with the heaven-qi and earth-qi.

3. 通调龙火两路

3.3　To regulate the dragon and fire channels

人体内存在着两条极为重要的内封闭道路，即龙路和火路，龙路、火路构成网络，在人体体表密布网结，这些网结即为穴位。人体"嘘"（气）、"勒"（血）、精水等营养物质通过龙路火路的输布滋养脏腑骨肉。同时龙路、火路也是邪毒内侵的主要途径。壮医药浴疗法直接作用于龙路、火路在体表的网结，疏通龙路、火路之瘀滞。一方面直接祛毒外出，另一方面，调整"嘘""勒"及脏腑功能，恢复天、人、地三气同步运行，从而达到治病的目的。

As two extremely important closed paths in the human body, the dragon and fire channels form a network on the body superficies. Their intersections are acupoints. Qi ("Xu" in the Zhuang language), blood ("Le" in the Zhuang language) and essence are transported via these two channels to nourish internal organs, bones and flesh. On the other hand, pathogenic toxins attack the body via these two channels. The ZM medicated bath therapy enables medicine to directly act on the acupoints to remove qi stagnation and blood stasis in the channels. Consequently, toxins can be removed, and qi, blood and the functions of zang-fu organs can be regulated, resulting in restoration of the synchronization of the heaven-qi, earth-qi and human-qi. Ultimately, diseases can be cured.

二、技法特色
Ⅱ Characteristics of the therapy

（一）理论特色
1 Theoretical features

壮医认为人体健康状态归结于"通""动""衡"，"通"即三道两路（谷道、水道、气道、龙路、火路）通畅，"动"即天、地、人三部之气协调同步运行，"衡"即气血阴阳平衡。气血失衡是疾病发生发展的根源。龙路相当于人体的血管，是血液循环的枢纽和通路；火路相当于人体的大脑和神经，是信息传导感应的通路。壮医认为，各种毒邪蕴积于肌表，使龙路、火路网络阻滞不通，气血失衡，三气不能同步；或体质素虚，脏腑功能不调，毒邪内生，进而导致疾病的发生。

From the perspective of ZM, body health is maintained by "smoothness", "movement" and "balance". Specifically, "smoothness" means the three passages and two channels (i.e. the grain, water and qi passages, and the dragon and fire channels) are unobstructed; "movement" refers to the synchronization of the heaven-qi, earth-qi and human-qi; and "balance" means the balance between qi and blood, the balance between yin and yang. Imbalance between qi and blood is the root cause for onset and development of a disease. In ZM, the dragon channel refers to the blood vessels, which are the hub and pathway of blood circulation; and the fire channel refers to the brain and nervous system, through which information is conducted. Retention of toxic pathogens on the body superficies blocks the dragon and fire channels, leading to an imbalance between qi and blood, and the failure of synchronization of three kinds of qi. This ultimately results in diseases. ZM also thinks diseases can be caused by the toxic pathogens internally produced due to congenitally weak constitution and dysfunction of zang-fu organs.

皮肤官窍为邪气侵入人体的必经之路，壮医药浴疗法借助热力配合药力作用于人体肌表，以疏通龙路、火路，调节天、地、人三气的同步平衡，达到疗疾养生的目的。

The orifices of the skin are the only ways for pathogenic qi to invade the human body. The ZM medicated bath therapy makes use of the synergistic effect of heat and medicine on the body superficies to unblock the dragon and fire channels and make the heaven-qi, earth-qi and human-qi synchronized, finally resulting in treatment of disease and health care.

（二）临床特色
2　Clinical features

1. 患者易于接受
2.1　High acceptance rate

壮医药浴疗法一般只需选用临床常用的中草药，加工制成所需剂型，通过熏、洗、浴、浸、渍等方法用药，药切皮肤，即可达到防病治病的目的。该疗法既可避免打针之痛、吃药之苦，又为治病提供新的给药途径，可以弥补内治法的不足。

In the ZM medicated bath therapy, commonly used Chinese medical herbs directly act on the skin in various modes, such as steaming, washing, bathing and soaking, to treat and prevent diseases. This therapy enables patients not to withstand pain caused by injection and oral administration of medicine. Therefore, it can be regarded as an alternative solution to the problems that internal treatment methods cannot resolve.

2. 减少药物破坏

2.2　Reduction of side effects

药物外用，不经消化道吸收，可以避免各种消化酶和肝脏代谢功能对药效的影响。

When medicines are used externally, they will not be absorbed through the digestive tract, which cannot be influenced by various digestive enzymes and liver metabolism.

3. 用药安全灵活

2.3　Safety and flexibility

壮医药浴疗法从体外施药，可以减少对消化道的刺激和对肝脏的损害，比口服用药更加安全可靠；可随时停用；方法简单，便于应用，患者自己可以操作。

The ZM medicated bath therapy reduces irritation to the digestive tract and damage to the liver because medicines are externally used. Therefore, to a large extent, it is safer and more reliable than oral administration of medicine. It can stop being used at any time. Its procedure is so simple that patients can easily use it on their own.

4. 适用范围广

2.4　A wide range of indications

壮医药浴疗法不仅适用于外科疾病，如疮疡肿毒、跌打损伤和皮肤病，而且可广泛用于内科、妇科、儿科、五官科等科的疾病。

The ZM medicated bath therapy is applicable in external medical conditions, including sores, ulcers, swelling, injury from knocks and falls, and skin diseases. It can also be used to treat internal medical conditions such as internal, gynecological, pediatric and ENT diseases.

5. 药源广泛易得

2.5　Easy access to Zhuang herbal medicinals

壮医药浴疗法用药以壮族地区道地药材为主，而广西、广东、云南等壮族地区素来药用资源丰富，药材易于收集。

Herbal medicinals used in the ZM medicated bath therapy are normally gathered in the regions where the Zhuang people live. Such regions in Guangxi, Guangdong and Yunnan are well known for exuberant medical resources, so medicinals needed are readily available.

6. 操作简便

2.6　Simple operation

壮医药浴疗法只需使用到锅具、盆具等家居用品，通过将壮药材进行简易加工即可施治，易于掌握、运用与推广。

The ZM medicated bath therapy can be easily applied and promoted because it only needs household items such as a pot to boil medicinals with water and a basin to hold the decoction.

（三）选药特色

3　Features of herbal medicinal selection

1. 喜用生药

3.1　Preference for raw herbal medicinals

壮族地区草木繁茂，四季常青，拥有丰富的动植物资源，具备使用新鲜药物的环境和条件，故壮医形成了使用生药的习惯。生药未经干燥、加工等环节，有效成分丢失较少，因而疗效比干品或炮制品更好。

The areas where the Zhuang people live are covered with lush evergreen vegetation and have abundance of plant and animal resources, which makes fresh herbal medicinals readily accessible. This enables ZM practitioners to use raw herbal medicinals as they like. Compared with dried and processed herbal medicinals, the curative effect of raw ones is better because more active ingredients in them are preserved.

不少民间壮医能从生草药的形态性味大抵推测出其功能作用，并将用药经验编成歌诀，以便于吟诵和传授，如"藤木通心定祛风，对枝对叶可除红；枝叶有刺能消肿，叶里藏浆拔毒功；辛香定痛驱寒湿，甘味滋补虚弱用；圆梗白花寒性药，热药梗方花色红；根黄清热退黄用，节大跌打驳骨雄；苦能解毒兼清热，咸寒降下把坚攻；味淡多为利水药，酸涩收敛涤污脓"等。使用动物药的规律为"虫类祛风止痛定惊，鳞类化瘀散结，飞禽走兽滋补气血"等。

Many ZM practitioners can infer the usage of raw herbal medicinals by observing their shapes, and recognizing their natures and tastes. Besides, they imparted their experience of medication by compiling them into verses which can be easily recited. For example, empty vines are used to dispel wind; tree branches and leaves growing in juxtaposition are used to reduce redness; branches and leaves with thorn are used to remove swelling; leaves containing pulp are used to draw out toxins; vegetation with spicy taste and pleasant smell is used to relieve pain and remove cold and dampness; vegetation with sweet taste is used to reinforce deficiency; round stems and white flowers are cold in nature; square stems and red flowers are heat in nature; yellow stems are used to clear away heat and eliminate jaundice; large branches are used to treat injury from knocks and falls and set fractured bones; vegetation with bitter taste is used to remove toxins and clear away heat; vegetation with salty taste is used to remove cold and soften lumps; vegetation with light taste is often used to induce diuresis; vegetation with sour and astringent taste is used to arrest discharge and flush pus away; insects are used to dispel wind, relieve pain and arrest convulsion; the squamata are used to remove blood stasis and dissipate nodules; and birds and beasts are used to tonify qi and blood.

2. 辨病为主，专方专药

3.2　Dedicated formula for treatment of specific disease based on syndrome differentiation

壮医药浴疗法以辨病为主，多主张针对不同的病因、不同的疾病选用专病专药。

Based on syndrome differentiation, different herbal medicinals are used in the ZM medicated bath therapy to treat diseases with different causes.

临床上应用的壮医方药，有不少是根据几千年的临床实践总结出来的专病专方。数千年来，在广大壮族民众聚居地区，民间流传着非常丰富的、组方简单而疗效神奇的治疗疑难杂症的偏方、秘方、验方。这些流传于民间的方剂有一个共同的特点——一个验方专治一种病，因此，称之为专病专方。专病专方的主要特点是药味不多，对某些病证具有独特疗效；流传于民间口口相授，一般医药古籍中多无收载，或仅见于民间医师的手抄本。

Many of ZM formulas used in present clinical practices are summarized based on thousands of years of experience in medical practices. For thousands of years, many special but irregular recipes, secret formulas and proven formulas circulate in the settlements of the Zhuang nationality. These formulas consist of simple medicinal substances but take remarkable efficacy on treatment of intractable diseases. They have it in common that a formula is dedicated to a specific disease, so they are known as "dedicated formula for treatment of specific disease". Such formulas are handed down by mouth of word or only found in the manuscripts of folk medical practitioners.

专病专方是顺应传统壮医辨病为主的基础理论，以及用药简便廉捷的临床特点而产生和发展的。典型的专病专方包括单味黄花蒿治疗疟疾、山芝麻配金银花治痧病、飞扬草治疗腹泻等。

The dedicated formulas are justified by the basic ZM principle of syndrome differentiation and treatment, and characterized by simplicity, convenience, low cost and quickness in operation. There are many popular dedicated formulas. For example, Huanghuahao (*Artemisia annua* Linn.) is used to treat malaria; the simple formula consisting of Shanzhima (Radix Helicteris Angustifoliae) and Jinyinhua (Flos Lonicerae) is used for filth; Feiyangcao (Herba Euphorbiae Hirtae) is used for diarrhea.

3. 对因治疗

3.3　Cause determination and treatment

壮医内治的重点是"因"和"病"。对因治疗就是指针对不同的疾病、不同的病因进行不同的治疗。壮医认为，人体生病，大多或为毒，或为虚所致。"毒""虚"致百病，有病必有因，对因治疗，实为治病求其本之意，病因一除，其病自会慢慢痊愈。例如壮医治疗瘴病，针对瘴毒选用青蒿、槟榔等；壮医治疗癌症，针对癌毒选用金银花、板蓝根、山芝麻、黄皮果等；壮医治疗瘀病，针对瘀毒选用田七、桃仁、赤芍等；壮医治疗疮肿，针对热毒、火毒选用两面针、半边莲、大青叶、七叶莲等；壮医治疗黄疸病，则针对湿热瘀毒选用茵陈、田基黄、郁金等。这些都是对因治疗的具体实例。

The treatment of internal diseases in ZM is focused on "causes" and "diseases".

In other words, treatment is based on determination of the cause of illness. Diseases are normally caused by toxins or deficiency. From the perspective of ZM, there must be a fundamental cause for a disease, and thus following the therapeutic principle of treating disease from the root cause can make a disease be cured. For example, for diseases caused by filth, use Qinghao (Herba Artemisiae Annuae) and Binglang (Semen Arecae) because they can remove filth; for cancers, use Jinyinhua (Flos Lonicerae), Banlangen (Radix Isatidis), Shanzhima (Radix Helicteris Angustifoliae) and Huangpiguo (Fruit of Chinese Wampee); for diseases caused by stasis, use Tianqi (Radix Notoginseng), Taoren (Semen Persicae) and Chishao (Radix Paeoniae Rubra); for sores and swelling, use Liangmianzhen (Radix Zanthoxyli), Banbianlian (Herba Lobeliae Chinensis), Daqingye (Folium Isatidis) and Qiyelian (Caulis et Folium Schefflerae Arboricolae) because they can clear away heat and fire; for jaundice, use Yinchen (Herba Artemisiae Scopariae), Tianjihuang (Herba Hyperici Japonici) and Yujin (Radix Curcumae).

4. 对症治疗

3.4　Treatment based on symptoms

壮医对症治疗，是对因治疗的补充。即在对因治疗治其本的基础上，针对不同的症状，选用一些药物以治其标，控制症状。如对于外感热毒证，咽痛者加毛冬青、鱼腥草、穿心莲、玉叶金花；咳嗽者加王瓜、十大功劳、三叉苦、百部、穿破石。对于某些疾病，有疼痛者加两面针、通城虎、金耳环、茉莉根、青药、山香皮、九里香等。总之，对症治疗就是针对主要症状或主要兼症进行治疗，对于具体病证而言，主要症状和兼症均需视具体情况而定。

Treating the incidental is supplementary to treating the radical. In other words, in addition to treating the radical, the manifestations of a diseases should be treated. For example, for a disease of which the root cause is heat, if the chief manifestation is pain in the throat, add Maodongqing (Radix Llicis Pubescentis), Yuxingcao (Herba Houttuyniae), Chuanxinlian (Herba Andrographis) and Yuyejinhua (Caulis et Radix Mussaendae Pubescentis); and if the chief manifestation is cough, add Wanggua (Fruit of Japanese Snakegourd), Shidagonglao (Folium Mahoniae), Sanchaku (Folium et Ramulus Evodiae Laptae), Baibu (Radix Stemonae) and Chuanposhi

(Radix Cudraniae Cochinchinensis); for some diseases accompanied by pain, add Liangmianzhen (Radix Zanthoxyli), Tongchenghu (Ovalleaf Dutchmanspipe Root), Jinerhuan (Herba Asarl Insignis), Moligen (Radix Jasmini Sambac), Qingyao (*Aster faberi* Franch.), Shanxiangpi (Cortex Hyptis Suaveolentis) and Jiulixiang (Folium et Cacumen Murrayae). In a word, treating the incidental refers to treating main symptoms and major complications, which are variable due to different medical conditions.

（四）浴种特色

4　Features of bathing

根据不同作用部位可选择不同药浴形式。

Different medicated bath methods are selected as appropriate.

1. 全身洗浴法

4.1　Whole-body bath

用壮药煎汤，将药汤倒入大盆或大木桶，待水温在 35 ℃左右时，令患者坐入盆（桶）中浸泡 20～30 分钟。适用于全身性疾病及养生保健。

Boil Zhuang herbal medicinals with water and pour the decoction into a large pot or a large wooden barrel. When the water temperature drops at 35 ℃, ask patients to soak for 20 to 30 minutes. It is suitable for diseases and health care in different parts of the whole body.

2. 局部浸洗法

4.2　Local bath

用壮药煎汤后倒入盆中，浸泡患者患部或手足部位，适用于局部性疾病及养生保健。

Boil Zhuang herbal medicinals with water and pour the decoction into a pot. When the water temperature is proper, ask patients to soak their disease sites, or hands and feet. It is suitable for diseases and health care in the affected area.

3. 坐浴法（坐盆法）

4.3　Hip bath (also known as sitz bath)

用壮药煎汤后倒入盆内，待水温为 35～40 ℃时，让患者坐进盆里。主治会阴部位疾病。

Boil Zhuang herbal medicinals with water and pour the decoction into a pot. When the water temperature drops at 35~40 ℃ , ask patients to sit in it to treat vaginal diseases.

4. 冲洗法

4.4 Washing

用壮药煎汤后倒入容器中，冲洗全身或局部，适用于不宜洗浴与坐浴的疾病及养生保健。

Boil Zhuang herbal medicinals with water and pour the decoction into a pot, and then ask patients to rinse their whole body or affected areas. It is used when the forementioned three methods are not suitable.

5. 擦洗法

4.5 Scrubbing

用壮药煎汤后倒入容器中，待温度约 40 ℃时擦洗患处。此法借助药力和摩擦力作用于患处，适用于以局部疾病为主的患者及行动不便者。

Boil Zhuang herbal medicinals with water and pour the decoction into a pot. When the water temperature drops at about 40 ℃ , ask patients to scrub the affected areas. It is suitable for those with lesion at a local area or reduced mobility.

三、操作规范
Ⅲ Specifications for operation

（一）前期准备
1 Pre-treatment preparation

1. 用物准备

1.1 Preparation of materials

治疗车、清洁治疗盘、阳证或阴证壮药液及药包、一次性药浴袋、手套2 副、浴巾 1 张、毛巾 2 张、病人服 1 套、拖鞋、水温计、手电筒、温开水、手消毒液、钟表、治疗单、笔、垃圾桶（图 19 ）。

A treatment cart, a treatment pad, bags of decoction for yin or yang syndrome, disposable plastic bags, two pairs of gloves, a bath towel, two towels, a set of patient clothes, a pair of slippers, a thermometer, a flashlight, warm water, hand sanitizer, a clock/watch, medication sheets, a pen and trash cans (Fig. 19).

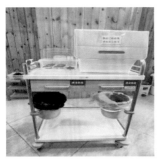 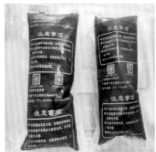 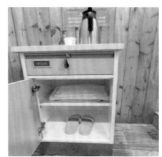

图 19　用物准备

Fig. 19　Preparation of materials

2. 药浴室环境准备

1.2　Preparation of a bathroom

浴缸、椅子、排气装置、供暖系统、供水系统（图 20）。

A bathtub, chairs, an exhaust, a heating system, a water supply (Fig. 20).

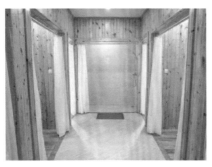 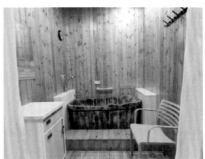

图 20　药浴室环境准备

Fig. 20　Preparation of a bathroom

（二）操作流程

2　Operating procedure

（1）双人核对医嘱、治疗单。评估患者，洗手，戴口罩。

(1) Cross-check the instructions for the therapy and medication sheets, evaluate the patient's medical conditions, wash the hands and wear a mask.

（2）打开浴室排气扇，调节室内温度为 24 ～ 28 ℃，将一次性药浴袋套入清洁浴缸，加入 40 ℃温水至浴缸的 1/2 ～ 2/3，将壮药药液倒入浴缸内与温水混合，测量药液温度，以 37 ～ 42 ℃为宜（图 21）。

(2) Turn on the bathroom exhaust fan and set the room temperature between 24 and 28 ℃, wrap the bathtub with a disposable plastic bag and fill it with water at 40 ℃ to be 1/2 or 2/3 full, pour the decoction into the bathtub and adjust the water temperature to be 37 to 42 ℃ (Fig. 21).

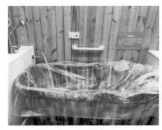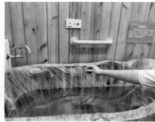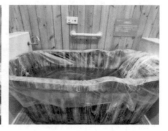

图 21　准备药液
Fig. 21　Preparation of the decoction

（3）核对患者床号、姓名、年龄、治疗部位等信息，指引患者至药浴室。

(3) Check the patient's bed number, name, age and applied areas, and take the patient to the bathroom.

（4）入浴。指导患者入浴，协助褪去衣物，进入浴缸，取坐位或舒适体位。

(4) Help the patient to take off their clothes, instruct them to enter the tub and take the sitting position or find another proper position for soaking.

（5）泡浴。水位以至患者胸部以下为宜。指导患者用毛巾不断将药液淋洗至上身。泡浴约 5 分钟后根据患者的耐受程度调整水温，以达到最佳效果。患者头面部、全身皮肤微红，有轻微汗出属正常治疗效果，予及时擦汗，指导患者多饮温开水。泡浴时间为 15 ～ 30 分钟。

(5) Keep the water level below the patient's chest and ask the patient to rinse their body above the chest with a decoction-soaked towel. Five minutes later, adjust the water temperature based on the patient's tolerance to heat to achieve the optimal

efficacy of medicine. It is normal if the skin of the head, face and whole body is slightly reddened with sweat. Advise the patient to wipe sweat in time and drink more warm water. Normally, leave them to soak for about 15 to 30 minutes.

（6）观察。

①注意测量药液温度，以患者轻微汗出、耐受为宜。

②观察患者面色、呼吸、局部皮肤情况，询问患者的感受，避免患者虚脱。

(6) During soaking, keep the water temperature hot enough to make the patient slightly sweat but able to withstand the heat. Observe their complexion, breath rate, skin condition on the local area and check their feelings from time to time to prevent heat syncope from happening.

（7）起浴。

①指导患者清洁，擦干头发及皮肤，协助患者穿衣。

②询问患者对操作的感受。

③指导患者：起浴后皮肤表面发红，有轻微的头晕、乏力及持续 30 分钟至 1 个小时的发汗均属正常的药效反应，应卧床休息 1 ～ 2 小时，不可吹风，注意保暖，及时更衣；起浴后应适当补充水分，忌食生冷、油腻、寒凉及酸辣刺激之品，可服用壮医药膳及茶饮。

(7) Instruct the patient to clean up and dry off their hair and body and assist them in dressing. Then check their feelings about bathing. Tell them it is normal if their skin is reddened, they feel slightly lightheaded and fatigue, or sweating lasts for 30 minutes to 1 hour. Advise them to rest in bed for 1~2 hours, avoid wind, keep themselves warm, put on clean dry clothes. After bathing, advise them to drink some water, Zhuang herbal medicinal soup or tea and avoid uncooked, cold, greasy, sour, spicy and stimulating foods.

（8）再次核对患者信息，致谢。

(8) Check the patient's information again and thank the patient for their cooperation.

（9）洗手，记录。

(9) Wash the hands and make a post-operative record.

（10）按消毒技术规范要求分类整理使用后的物品。

(10) Sort out the used devices according to the disinfection technical specifications.

（三）注意事项

3　Cautions

（1）泡洗药液温度不宜过高，以防烫伤，老年人、感觉迟钝者的泡洗温度不宜超过 38 ℃。

(1) Do not make the water temperature too high to avoid scalding burns. For the elderly people and those who are not sensitive to heat, keep it no higher than 38 ℃.

（2）所用物品须清洁消毒，物品一人一份一消毒，避免交叉感染。

(2) Clean and disinfect all items. Use one set of items on one patient to prevent cross infection.

（3）药浴过程中若患者出现头晕、胸闷、心悸、全身乏力等症状，立即停止药浴，进行急救。

(3) Stop soaking and perform first aid if symptoms occur, including dizziness, chest stuffiness, palpitation and malaise.

（4）女性处于月经期及妊娠期时禁用此疗法。

(4) Never apply the ZM medicated bath therapy to those during menstruation or pregnancy.

四、常见病证治疗

Ⅳ　Treatment of common diseases

（一）年闹诺（失眠）

1　Insomnia ("Niannaonuo" in ZM)

1. 疾病概述

1.1　General description

年闹诺指经常不能获得正常睡眠的一种疾病，临床病情轻重不一。轻者主要表现为入睡困难，或睡中易醒，或醒后不能再睡；重者彻夜难眠，常伴有神疲乏力、头晕头痛、健忘或心神不宁等症。本病临床较常见，多为情志失调、久病体弱、饮食不节、劳逸失度等引起。

"Niannaonuo" refers to sleep disorders, of which the clinical manifestations differ. The symptoms of mild insomnia include difficulty falling asleep at night, waking up during the night and inability to sleep after waking up. Severe insomnia is characterized by inability to sleep throughout the night, often accompanied by lassitude, dizziness, headache, forgetfulness or restlessness. The disorders are often caused by excessive emotion activities, weak constitution due to long-term illness, dietary irregularities and imbalance between work and rest.

年闹诺相当于中医的不寐、不得眠、不得卧、目不瞑；西医的神经衰弱综合征、失眠亦可参考本病进行诊治。

"Niannaonuo" is the same as sleeplessness or inability to sleep in TCM, and neurasthenia or insomnia in WM, so the treatment of these medical conditions can refer to that of "Niannaonuo".

2. 病因病机

1.2　Cause and mechanism of disease

壮医认为，年闹诺发生的原因主要有以下几点。

From the perspective of ZM, there are three main causes of insomnia.

（1）情志失调，思虑过度，恼怒太过，情志不舒，致体内脏腑气机郁滞，阴阳失调，天、地、人三气不能同步。

(1) Excessive emotional activities such as pensiveness and anger cause depression and stagnation of qi movement in zang-fu organs, leading to the imbalance between yin and yang. Consequently, the human-qi fails to synchronize itself with the heaven-qi and earth-qi.

（2）先天禀赋不足，后天失养，或房劳过度，肾精亏损，或劳累太过，大病之后失于调理，致气血不足，心虚胆怯，阴阳失调，天、地、人三气不能同步。

(2) Congenital defect combined with lack of proper postnatal care, kidney essence deficiency due to excess of sexual activity, overexertion, or lack of proper care after illness, can cause the deficiency of qi and blood, and heart deficiency with

gallbladder timidity. This leads to the imbalance between yin and yang, resulting in failure of synchronization of the heaven-qi, earth-qi and human-qi.

（3）饮食不节，过饥过饱，或过食辛辣、生冷、油腻之品，热毒、痰毒等邪毒内生，气机不畅，胃气不和，致阴阳失调，天、地、人三气不能同步。

(3) Dietary irregularities, such as overeating or extreme hunger and overeating spicy, uncooked, cold or greasy foods, will make heat and phlegm internally produced, resulting in stagnation of qi movement and stomach qi disharmony. This will lead to the imbalance between yin and yang, and thus the human-qi fails to synchronize itself with the heaven-qi and earth-qi.

总之，不能获得正常睡眠的原因很多，有思虑劳倦，七情内伤，心肝火旺，胃失和降，使心神被扰或气血两虚，伤及心和"味隆"（脾），生血之源不足，巧坞失养所致；或惊悉、房劳伤及"咪腰"（肾），以致心火独炽，心肾不交，阴阳不调，神志不宁。

In a word, there are many causes of sleep disorders. For example, one cause is that the brain does not obtain enough nutrients. Mental exhaustion, internal injuries caused by seven emotions, hyperactivity of the heart-fire and liver-fire, and failure of stomach qi to descend can lead to mental disturbance or the dual deficiency of qi and blood. This will cause damage to the heart and spleen ("Weilong" in the Zhuang language) where blood is produced, leading to insufficiency of blood. As a result, nutrients transported by blood to the brain will be not adequate, resulting in the inadequate nourishment of the brain. Another cause can be restlessness. When the kidney ("Miyao" in the Zhuang language) is injured due to fright and sexual consumption, hyperactivity of the heart-fire and disharmony of the heart and kidney will occur. This will cause the imbalance between yin and yang and the mind restless.

3. 诊查要点

1.3　Essentials for diagnosis

（1）诊断依据。

(1) Diagnosis criteria.

① 主症。久久不能入睡，或睡而不稳反复醒来，或早醒不能再睡，或时睡时醒，甚至彻夜不能入睡。

① Main symptoms: Inability to fall asleep soon, sleep instability with recurrent wake-up, early morning waking with inability to sleep again, mid-sleep awakening, or inability to be asleep all night.

② 兼症。头重头痛，急躁易怒，眼红口苦，小便黄，大便秘结，舌下脉络粗胀，色青紫，口唇绛红；或心烦，头晕耳鸣，健忘，脸色少华等。

② Concurrent symptoms: Heavy sensation in the head, headache, irritability, red eyes, bitter taste in the mouth, yellow urine, constipation, enlarged bluish purple blood vessels on the lower surface of the tongue, crimson red lips, or vexation, dizziness, tinnitus, forgetfulness and lusterless complexion.

③ 甲诊。指甲颜色鲜红或淡白，半月痕暴露过多或过少，或按压指尖后放开，久久未恢复红润，指甲呈紫赤甲、横沟甲、竹笋甲或葱管甲等。

③ Nail examination: Fingernails are bright red or pale with small or large fingernail lunulae. When a fingernail stops being pressed, the color of the fingernail will return slowly. There are red-purple dots or Beau's lines on the nail bed, or the nail looks like bamboo shoot or scallion.

④ 目诊。勒答白睛上脉络弯曲多，弯度大，脉络多而集中，靠近瞳仁；或勒答白睛上脉络弯曲少，弯度小，颜色较浅，脉络分散。

④ Eye examination: Many large-radius bends are on the blood vessels of the white of the eyes, many of which are visible and close to the pupils; or a few small-radius bends are on the blood vessels of the white of the eyes, which are reddish and scattered.

（2）病证鉴别。

(2) Symptom differentiation.

① 一过性失眠：在日常生活中常见，可为一时性情志不舒，生活环境改变，或饮用浓茶、咖啡和服用药物等引起。一般有明显诱因，且病程不长。一过性失眠不属病态，也不用进行任何治疗，可通过身体自然调节而复常。

① Transient insomnia: As a common sleep disturbance, it is caused by apparent reasons, including short-term emotional disorder, life change, strong tea and coffee consumption, and medication taking. It does not last very long. It is not pathological and is usually self-resolved.

② 生理性少寐：多见于老年人，虽少寐早醒，但无明显痛苦，属生理现象。

② Physiological insomnia: It occurs primarily in the elderly people. It is characterized by reduced sleep quantity and early morning waking but without obvious pain, so it is a physiological phenomenon.

4. 辨证论治

1.4　Syndrome differentiation and treatment

（1）治疗原则。平衡气血，调理气机。

(1) Treatment principles. Harmonize qi with blood and adjust qi movement.

（2）证治分类。

(2) Classification of syndrome identification and treatment.

① 阳证。心烦不能入睡，烦躁易怒，胸闷胁痛，头痛面红，目赤，便秘尿黄，胸闷脘痞，口苦痰多，头晕目眩。舌红，苔黄或黄腻，脉大、急、有力。

① Yang syndrome. Inability to sleep due to vexation, irritability, chest stuffiness, hypochondriac pain, headache, flushed face with crimson eyes, constipation, yellow urine, stomach cavity stuffiness, bitter taste in the mouth with much sputum, dizziness, blurred vision, red tongue with yellow or yellow, greasy coating, and large, rapid forceful pulse.

治疗原则：解毒，调气。

Treatment principles: Remove toxins and adjust qi.

选药：鬼针草、夜交藤、合欢皮、龙骨、牡蛎、九龙藤。

Prescription: Guizhencao (Herba Bidentis Pilosae), Yejiaoteng (Caulis Polygoni Multiflori), Hehuanpi (Cortex Albiziae), Longgu (Os Draconis), Muli (Concha Ostreae) and Jiulongteng (Radix seu Caulis Bauhiniae Championii).

如热毒盛，可选用淡竹叶、半枝莲、黄芩、路边菊、连钱草；痰毒盛，可选用石菖蒲、陈皮、火炭母、夏枯草；湿毒盛，可选用蒲公英、垂盆草、虎杖、六月雪、五加皮；气郁重，可选用钩藤、薄荷、萝芙木、含羞草、荔枝核；血瘀重，可选用土牛膝、鹰不扑、艾叶、侧柏叶、墨旱莲、苏木。

For those with severe heat, add Danzhuye (Herba Lophatheri), Banzhilian (Herba Scutellariae Barbatae), Huangcen (Radix Scutellariae), Lubianju (Herba Kalimeridis Indicae) and Lianqiancao (Herba Glechomae); for those with severe phlegm, add

Shichangpu (Rhizoma Acori Tatarinowii), Chenpi (Pericarpium Citri Reticulatae), Huotanmu (Herba Polygoni Chinensis) and Xiakucao (Spica Prunellae); for those with exuberant dampness, add Pugongying (Herba Taraxaci), Chuipencao (Herba Sedi Sarmentosi), Huzhang (Rhizoma et Radix Polygoni Cuspidati), Liuyuexue (Herba Serissae) and Wujiapi (Cortex Acanthopanacis); for those with severe qi depression, add Gouteng (Ramulus Uncariae cum Uncis), Bohe (Herba Menthae), Luofumu (Radix et Caulis Rauvolfiae), Hanxiucao (Herba Mimosae Pudicae) and Lizhihe (Semen Litchi); for those with severe blood stasis, add Tuniuxi (Radix et Rhizoma Achyranthis Asperae), Yingbupu (Radix Araliae Armatae), Aiye (Folium Artemisiae Argyi), Cebaiye (Cacumen Platycladi), Mohanlian (Herba Ecliptae) and Sumu (Lignum Sappan).

②阴证。中途易醒，醒后神疲乏力，胸闷胁痛，胸闷脘痞，痰多，心悸，头晕目眩；舌红，苔厚腻，脉大、滑、有力。

② Yin syndrome. Mid-sleep awakening with lassitude, chest stuffiness, hypochondriac pain, stomach cavity stuffiness, much sputum, palpitation, dizziness, blurred vision, red tongue with thick, greasy coating, and large, slippery forceful pulse.

治疗原则：解毒，调理气血。

Treatment principles: Remove toxins, and regulate qi and blood.

选药：佩兰、白芷、黑老虎、肿节风、桂枝、葛根、藿香。

Prescription: Peilan (Herba Eupatorii), Baizhi (Radix Angelicae Dahuricae), Heilaohu (Radix et Caulis Kadsurae Coccineae), Zhongjiefeng (Herba Sarcandrae), Guizhi (Ramulus Cinnamomi), Gegen (Radix Puerariae) and Huoxiang (Herba Agastaches).

如痰毒盛，可选用石菖蒲、陈皮、火炭母、夏枯草；湿毒盛，可选用蒲公英、垂盆草、虎杖、六月雪、生姜；气郁重，可选用钩藤、薄荷、萝芙木、含羞草、荔枝核、龙骨、牡蛎；血瘀重，可选用益母草、土牛膝、鹰不扑、艾叶、侧柏叶、墨旱莲、苏木、九龙藤。

For those with severe phlegm, add Shichangpu (Rhizoma Acori Tata-rinowii), Chenpi (Pericarpium Citri Reticulatae), Huotanmu (Herba Polygoni Chinensis) and Xiakucao (Spica Prunellae); for those with severe dampness, add Pugongying (Herba Taraxaci), Chuipencao (Herba Sedi Sarmentosi), Huzhang (Rhizoma et Radix Polygoni Cuspidati), Liuyuexue (Herba Serissae) and Shengjiang (Rhizoma Zingiberis Recens); for those with severe qi depression, add Gouteng (Ramulus Uncariae cum Uncis), Bohe (Herba Menthae), Luofumu (Radix et Caulis Rauvolfiae), Hanxiucao (Herba Mimosae Pudicae), Lizhihe (Semen Litchi), Longgu (Os Draconis) and Muli (Concha Ostreae); for those with severe blood stasis, add Yimucao (Herba Leonuri), Tuniuxi (Radix et Rhizoma Achyranthis Asperae), Yingbupu (Radix Araliae Armatae), Aiye (Folium Artemisiae Argyi), Cebaiye (Cacumen Platycladi), Mohanlian (Herba Ecliptae) Sumu (Lignum Sappan) and Jiulongteng (Radix seu Caulis Bauhiniae Championii).

③气血虚证。多梦易醒或浅睡不实，心悸，健忘，头晕目眩，神疲乏力，面色不华，多梦易惊，心悸胆怯；舌淡，苔薄，脉小、无力。

③ Qi and blood deficiency syndrome. Profuse dreaming with restless sleep or shallow sleep, palpitation, forgetfulness, dizziness, blurred vision, lassitude, lusterless complexion, profuse dreaming with susceptibility to fright, palpitation with gallbladder timidity, pale tongue with thin coating, and small, deep weak pulse.

治疗原则：补虚，调理气血。

Treatment principles: Reinforce deficiency, and regulate qi and blood.

选药：艾叶、五指毛桃、黄花倒水莲、杠板归、扶芳藤、路边菊、生姜、香茅。血虚，可选用土人参、鸡血藤、当归藤；气虚可选用墨旱莲、女贞子、夜交藤、合欢皮、五加皮、五指毛桃；气道虚，可选用龙利叶、仙鹤草、百部、牛大力；谷道病，可选用绞股蓝、牛大力、黄精；水道病，可选用巴戟天、骨碎补、狗脊、仙茅、千斤拔。

Prescription: Aiye (Folium Artemisiae Argyi), Wuzhimaotao (Radix Fici Hirtae), Huanghuadaoshuilian (Radix seu Folium Polygalae Fallacis), Gangbangui (Herba Polygoni Perfoliati), Fufangteng (Caulis Euonymi Fortunei cum Foliis), Lubianju (Herba Kalimeridis Indicae), Shengjiang (Rhizoma Zingiberis Recens) and Xiangmao (Herba Cymbopogonis Citrari).

For those with blood deficiency, add Turenshen (Radix Talini Paniculati),

Jixueteng (Caulis Spatholobi) and Dangguiteng (*Embelia Parviflora* Wall.); for those with qi deficiency, add Mohanlian (Herba Ecliptae), Nvzhenzi (Fructus Ligustri Lucidi), Yejiaoteng (Caulis Polygoni Multiflori), Hehuanpi (Cortex Albiziae) and Wujiapi (Cortex Acanthopanacis) and Wuzhimaotao (Radix Fici Hirtae); for those with qi passage deficiency, add Longliye (Folium Sauropi), Xianhecao (Herba Agrimoniae), Baibu (Radix Stemonae) and Niudali (Radix Millettiae Speciosae); for those with diseases occurs in the grain passage, add Jiaogulan (Herba Gynostemmatis Pentaphylli), Niudali (Radix Millettiae Speciosae) and Huangjing (Rhizonma Polygonati); for those with diseases occurs in the water passage, add Bajitian (Radix Morindae Officinalis), Gusuibu (Rhizoma Drynariae), Gouji (Rhizoma Cibotii), Xianmao (Rhizoma Curculiginis) and Qianjinba (Radix et Caulis Flemingiae).

5. 预防调护

1.5　Prevention and care

年闹诺属心神病变，重视精神调摄和讲究睡眠卫生对该病具有实际的预防意义。积极进行心理情志调整，克服过度的紧张、兴奋、焦虑、抑郁、惊恐、愤怒等不良情绪，做到喜怒有节，保持精神舒畅，尽量以放松的、顺其自然的心态对待睡眠，反而能较好地入睡。

From the perspective of ZM, insomnia is a type of pathological changes in the heart and mind. It can be prevented by paying close attention to mind adjustment and sleep hygiene. It can be overcome by making psychological and emotional adjustment and avoiding excessive emotional activities such as nervousness, excitement, anxiety, depression, fright and anger. Keeping the spirit up and keeping the mind relaxed are helpful to falling asleep.

在对年闹诺患者的护理上，首先要帮助患者建立有规律的作息制度，令其进行适当的体力活动或体育锻炼，增强体质，持之以恒，以促进身心健康。其次要让患者养成良好的睡眠习惯。晚餐要清淡，不宜过饱，更忌饮浓茶、咖啡及吸烟。睡前避免从事紧张和兴奋的活动，养成定时就寝的习惯。另外，要注意睡眠环境的安宁，床铺要舒适，卧室光线要柔和，并努力减少噪声，去除各种可能影响睡眠的外在因素。

In term of insomnia nursing care, provide patients with the following advice.

First, establish a regular life schedule and advise them to engage in appropriate physical activities or work out regularly and properly to strengthen the body and promote physical and mental health. Second, develop and maintain good sleep habits, for example, having a light dinner, avoiding alcohol or coffee consumption, smoking as well as stressful or exciting activities before sleep, and going to bed at the same time every day. Third, create a good sleep environment. Specifically, reduce noise as much as possible to keep the environment quiet, make a comfortable bed, create soft lighting in the bedroom and attempt to eliminate external factors affecting sleep.

6. 医案选读

1.6　Selected case readings

【病案一】

［Case 1］

许某，男，30岁，2020年5月16日初诊。

Patient: Xu, a 30-year-old man, his first visit was on May 16, 2020.

主诉：失眠1月余。

Chief complaint:"I have had insomnia for more than 1 month."

现病史：患者最近1个多月来，因家庭及工作压力出现失眠，耗时1小时都难以入睡，易醒，醒后难入睡，伴口干口苦，急躁易怒，纳、寐可，二便正常。舌边及舌尖红，舌苔薄黄（图22），脉弦滑。

History of present illness: The patient reported difficulty falling asleep in the past month due to family-and work-related stress, inability to fall asleep within an hour, liability to waking up during night, inability to sleep after waking up, bitter taste in the mouth, thirst, irritability, good appetite, restful sleep, normal urination frequency and regular bowel movements. The tip and edges of his tongue are red with yellow (Fig. 22), thin coating. His pulse is wiry and slippery.

目诊：双侧白睛脉络鲜红。甲诊：指甲色泽红润，月痕偏大。壮医诊断：年闹诺（阳证）。中医诊断：不寐。西医诊断：失眠。

Eye examination: The blood vessels on the white of the eyes are bright red.

Nail examination: The nails are red with slightly large fingernail lunulae.

Diagnosis in ZM:"Niannaonuo" characterized by yang syndrome.

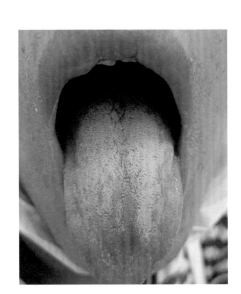

图 22　年闹诺（阳证）

Fig.22　"Niannaonuo" (yang syndrome)

Diagnosis in TCM: Sleeplessness.

Diagnosis in WM: Insomnia.

治疗原则：清热毒，畅气郁。

Treatment principles: Clear away heat and relieve qi depression.

治疗：壮医药浴疗法。

Treatment method: The ZM medicated bath therapy.

处方：鬼针草 30 g、夜交藤 30 g、合欢皮 30 g、九龙藤 30 g、路边菊 30 g、龙骨 30 g、牡蛎 30 g、五加皮 30 g、黄芩 30 g。7 次，每日 1 次。

Prescription: Guizhencao (Herba Bidentis Pilosae) 30 g, Yejiaoteng (Caulis Polygoni Multiflori) 30 g, Hehuanpi (Cortex Albiziae) 30 g, Jiulongteng (Radix seu Caulis Bauhiniae Championii) 30 g, Lubianju (Herba Kalimeridis Indicae) 30 g, Longgu (Os Draconis) 30 g, Muli (Concha Ostreae) 30 g, Wujiapi (Cortex Acanthopanacis) 30 g and Huangcen (Radix Scutellariae) 30 g. Take a bath daily for 7 days in a row.

二诊（2020 年 5 月 23 日）：经壮医药浴疗法治疗 7 次后，睡眠质量得到改善，能在半小时内入睡，时有夜间醒来，但醒后能快速入睡，已无口干口苦，二便正常，饮食佳，继予上方药浴治疗 5 次，巩固疗效。

Second visit (on May 23, 2020): After taking the ZM medicated bath seven times, the patient's sleep quality had been improved. He could fall asleep within half an hour. Although mid-sleep waking occurred, he could fall asleep again after awakening. He reported no bitter taste in the mouth, absence of thirst, good appetite, restful sleep, normal urination frequency and regular bowel movements. Accordingly, he was instructed to take the ZM medicated bath daily with the same prescription for another five days to consolidate the efficacy.

按语：本案患者失眠 1 月余，症见口干口苦，急躁易怒，脉弦滑，属阳证。乃思虑劳倦，七情内伤，热毒阻滞龙路、火路所致，治宜以泄火热之毒、通龙路火路为主。采用壮医药浴疗法治疗，药液中的鬼针草、夜交藤、合欢皮、路边菊、黄芩可畅气郁，五加皮、九龙藤行气除湿而通龙路、火路，可快速清泄体内火热之毒而畅通气机，热清则气血安和，火清则神安，则能寐矣。

Summary statement: The patient experienced insomnia for more than one month, which was manifested by bitter taste in mouth, thirst, irritability, and wiry, slippery pulse. These manifestations signified yang syndrome. Overthinking made him suffer from fatigue and emotional disorder, leading to emergence of heat. Subsequently, the heat blocked the dragon and fire channels. Therefore, the treatment principle was to clear away heat to unblock these two channels. In terms of the herbal medicinals used in the ZM medicated bath therapy, Guizhencao (Herba Bidentis Pilosae), Yejiaoteng (Caulis Polygoni Multiflori), Hehuanpi (Cortex Albiziae), Lubianju (Herba Kalimeridis Indicae) and Huangcen (Radix Scutellariae) were used to relieve qi depression; Wujiapi (Cortex Acanthopanacis) and Jiulongteng (Radix seu Caulis Bauhiniae Championii) were used to move qi and remove dampness to unblock the dragon and fire channels. In a word, quick removal of heat makes qi move. Clearing away heat can harmonize qi with blood, and thereby enable the mind to be restful, resulting in good sleep at night.

【病案二】

［Case 2］

韦某，男，38 岁，2020 年 9 月 28 日初诊。

Patient: Wei, a 38-year-old man, his first visit was on September 28, 2020.

主诉：失眠 1 月余。

Chief complaint:"I have had insomnia for more than 1 month."

现病史：患者述 1 个多月前无明显诱因下出现失眠，难以入睡，睡时多梦，睡中易醒，醒后神疲乏力，平素易胸闷心悸，头面有油腻感，无头晕头痛，无恶心欲吐等不适，纳、寐可，二便调。舌淡红，苔厚腻、润（图 23），脉弦滑。

History of present illness: The patient reported insomnia that occurred more than one month ago without any apparent reasons, inability to fall asleep, profuse dreaming with susceptibility to awakening, lassitude after waking up, chest stuffiness, palpitation, oily complexion, no dizziness, no headache, no nausea, good appetite, restful sleep, normal urination frequency and regular bowel movements. His tongue is reddish with thick, greasy and moist coating (Fig. 23). His pulse is wiry and slippery.

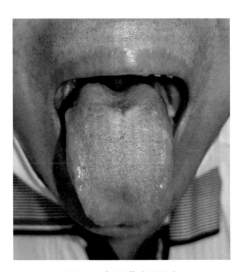

图 23　年闹诺（阴证）
Fig. 23 "Niannaonuo" (yin syndrome)

目诊：白睛色泽偏黄，少许脉络鲜红。甲诊：指甲淡红润泽。壮医诊断：年闹诺（阴证）。中医诊断：不寐。西医诊断：失眠。

Eye examination: The white of the eyes looks slightly yellow. A few blood vessels on the white of the eyes are bright red.

Nail examination: The nails are reddish and lustrous.

Diagnosis in ZM:"Niannaonuo" characterized by yin syndrome.

Diagnosis in TCM: Sleeplessness.

Diagnosis in WM: Insomnia.

治疗原则：除湿毒，调气血。

Treatment principles: Remove dampness and regulate qi and blood.

治疗：壮医药浴疗法。

Treatment method: The ZM medicated bath therapy.

处方：佩兰 30 g，白芷 30 g，益母草 30 g，黑老虎 30 g，肿节风 30 g，桂枝 15 g，葛根 30 g，藿香 30 g，生姜 30 g。7 次，隔日 1 次。

Prescription: Peilan (Herba Eupatorii) 30 g, Baizhi (Radix Angelicae Dahuricae) 30 g, Yimucao (Herba Leonuri) 30 g, Heilaohu (Radix et Caulis Kadsurae Coccineae) 30 g, Zhongjiefeng (Herba Sarcandrae) 30 g, Guizhi (Ramulus Cinnamomi) 30 g, Gegen (Radix Puerariae) 30 g, Huoxiang (Herba Agastaches) 30 g and Shengjiang (Rhizoma Zingiberis Recens) 30 g. Take the ZM medicated bath every two days, seven times in total.

二诊（2020 年 10 月 17 日）：经壮医药浴疗法治疗 7 次后，睡眠质量得到改善，易入睡，梦多情况明显减少，精力转佳，头面有油腻情况减轻，背部痤疮改善，心情愉悦。继续按原方案治疗 5 次，隔天 1 次，巩固疗效。

Second visit (on October 17, 2020): After taking the ZM medicated bath for seven times, The patient's sleep quality had been improved. Specifically, falling asleep became easier and dreamfulness was significantly reduced. Therefore, his energy was boosted, his complexion was less oily and the acne on his back was relieved. This made him be in a good mood. Accordingly, he was instructed to continue taking the ZM medicated bath with the same prescription every two days, five times in total, to consolidate the efficacy.

按语：本案患者失眠 1 月余，症见难以入睡，睡时多梦，睡中易醒，醒后神疲乏力，平素易胸闷心悸，头面有油腻感，舌淡红，苔厚腻、润，脉弦滑。属湿毒之阴证，治宜除湿以安神。采用壮医药浴疗法治疗，药液中的佩兰、白芷、桂枝、葛根、藿香、生姜除湿毒；益母草、黑老虎、肿节风活血通络。诸药合用可促进体内血液循环，使湿毒加快清除，共奏清泄体内湿毒，调三道之湿阻，通龙路、火路不畅之效，两路通，三道畅，自然神安助眠。

Summary statement: The patient experienced insomnia for more than one month. He reported inability to fall asleep, profuse dreaming with susceptibility to awakening, lassitude after waking up, chest stuffiness, palpitation and oily complexion. His tongue was reddish with thick, greasy and moist coating. His pulse was wiry and slippery. These manifestations signified yin syndrome of dampness. Therefore, the treatment principle was to remove dampness to calm the mind. In terms of the herbal medicinals used in the ZM medicated bath therapy, Peilan (Herba Eupatorii), Baizhi (Radix Angelicae Dahuricae), Guizhi (Ramulus Cinnamomi), Gegen (Radix Puerariae), Huoxiang (Herba Agastaches) and Shengjiang (Rhizoma Zingiberis Recens) were used to remove dampness; Yimucao (Herba Leonuri), Heilaohu (Radix et Caulis Kadsurae Coccineae) and Zhongjiefeng (Herba Sarcandrae) were used to activate blood and unblock the meridians. All the herbal medicinals combined had a synergistic effect to promote the blood circulation, expedite the removal of dampness, treat dampness impediment in the three passages and unblock the dragon and fire channels. As a result, the mind was restful and a good night's sleep was obtained.

【病案三】

［Case 3］

梁某，女，35 岁，2020 年 7 月 15 日初诊。

Patient: Liang, a 35-year-old woman, her first visit was on July 15, 2020.

主诉：反复失眠 6 个月。

Chief complaint:"I have had insomnia for six months."

现病史：患者最近 6 个月来无明显诱因下出现失眠，入睡困难，梦多，易醒，醒后难入睡，平素情绪波动，急躁易怒，经前乳房胀痛，神疲乏力，时有腰酸，纳、寐可，二便正常。舌淡红，舌苔薄白腻（图 24），脉弦细。

History of present illness: The patient has experienced insomnia in the past six months without any apparent reasons. She reported difficulty falling asleep, profuse dreaming with susceptibility to awakening, difficulty falling asleep again after waking up, frequent mood swings and irritability in daily life, breast pain before her menstruation, lassitude, occasional soreness in the lower back, good appetite, restful sleep, normal urination frequency and regular bowel movements. Her tongue is reddish with white (Fig. 24), thin coating. Her pulse is wiry and thready.

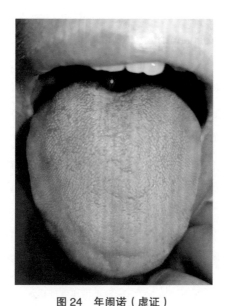

图 24 年闹诺（虚证）
Fig. 24 "Niannaonuo" (deficiency syndrome)

目诊：白睛脉络细小鲜红。甲诊：指甲色泽红润，甲体有少许细小竖条纹路。壮医诊断：年闹诺（虚证）。中医诊断：不寐。西医诊断：失眠。

Eye examination: The blood vessels on the white of the eyes are small and bright red.

Nail examination: There are a few narrow vertical stripes on the reddish and lustrous nails.

Diagnosis in ZM:"Niannaonuo" characterized by deficiency symptom.

Diagnosis in TCM: Sleeplessness.

Diagnosis in WM: Insomnia.

治疗原则：补虚，调和气血。

Treatment principles: Reinforce deficiency and harmonize qi and blood.

治疗：壮医药浴疗法。

Treatment method: The ZM medicated bath therapy.

处方：艾叶 50 g，五指毛桃 30 g，黄花倒水莲 30 g，杠板归 30 g，夜交藤 30 g，合欢皮 30 g，当归藤 30 g，路边菊 30 g，五加皮 30 g，扶芳藤 30 g，生姜 30 g，香茅 20 g。14 次，隔日 1 次。

Prescription: Aiye (Folium Artemisiae Argyi) 50 g, Wuzhimaotao (Radix Fici Hirtae) 30 g, Huanghuadaoshuilian (Radix seu Folium Polygalae Fallacis) 30 g, Gangbangui (Herba Polygoni Perfoliati) 30 g, Yejiaoteng (Caulis Polygoni Multiflori) 30 g, Hehuanpi (Cortex Albiziae) 30 g, Dangguiteng (*Embelia Parviflora* Wall.) 30 g, Lubianju (Herba Kalimeridis Indicae) 30 g, Wujiapi (Cortex Acanthopanacis) 30 g, Fufangteng (Caulis Euonymi Fortunei cum Foliis) 30 g, Shengjiang (Rhizoma Zingiberis Recens) 30 g and Xiangmao (Herba Cymbopogonis Citrari) 20 g. Take the ZM medicated bath every two days, fourteen times in total.

二诊（2020 年 7 月 30 日）：经壮医药浴疗法治疗 14 次后，睡眠质量明显改善，易入睡，梦多情况减少，虽时有夜间醒来，但醒后能快速入睡，精神精力转佳，已无明显腰酸乏力，二便正常，纳食佳，继续按原方案治疗 3 次，隔天 1 次，巩固疗效。

Second visit (on July 30, 2020): After taking the ZM medicated bath for fourteen times, the patient's sleep quality had been improved. Specifically, falling asleep became easier and dreamfulness was significantly reduced. Although mid-sleep awaking occurred, she could fall asleep soon after waking up. Therefore, her energy was boosted. Soreness in the lower back had disappeared. She reported good appetite, restful sleep, normal urination frequency and regular bowel movements. Accordingly, she was instructed to continue taking the ZM medicated bath with the same prescription every two days, three times in total, to consolidate the efficacy.

按语：本案患者失眠 6 个月，症见入睡困难，梦多，易醒。平素情绪波动、急躁易怒、经前乳房胀痛属阳证，同时伴有神疲乏力、腰酸、脉弦细为虚损不足之证。乃思虑劳倦，七情内伤，心肝火旺，胃失和降，使心神被扰或气血两虚，伤及心和"咪隆"（脾），生血之源不足，巧坞失养所致。治宜泄有余，补不足。采用壮医药浴疗法，药液中的夜交藤、合欢皮、当归藤、扶芳藤、五指毛桃、黄花倒水莲可补龙路火路之虚，五加皮、生姜、香茅、艾叶祛风毒、湿毒，杠板归利水道，路边菊解热毒。龙路火路网络遍布全身，而皮肤又为通调气道、水道的重要孔窍之一，药液经皮肤吸收，可通达龙路火路，再经气道、水道的气液交换，加快气血流通而畅达气机，诸药合用可泄体内有余之气热，补气血之不足，调整阴阳，睡眠可安。

Summary statement: The patient experienced insomnia for 6 months. She reported difficulty falling asleep, profuse dreaming with susceptibility to awakening, frequent mood swings, irritability, breast pain before her menstruation. These manifestations signified yang syndrome. Meanwhile, the symptoms, lassitude, soreness in the lower back and wiry, thready pulse, mean the yang syndrome was accompanied by consumption. Mental exhaustion, internal injuries caused by seven emotions, hyperactivity of the heart-fire and liver-fire, and/or failure of stomach qi to descend lead to mental disturbance or dual deficiency of qi and blood. As a result, the heart and spleen ("Weilong" in the Zhuang language), where blood is produced, were injured, leading to insufficiency of blood. Under such a circumstance, nutrients transported by blood to the brain were not adequate, resulting in the inadequate nourishment of the brain. Therefore, it was applicable to purge excess and reinforce deficiency. In terms of the herbal medicinals used in the ZM medicated bath therapy, Yejiaoteng (Caulis Polygoni Multiflori), Hehuanpi (Cortex Albiziae), Dangguiteng (*Embelia Parviflora* Wall.), Fufangteng (Caulis Euonymi Fortunei cum Foliis), Wuzhimaotao (Radix Fici Hirtae) and Huanghuadaoshuilian (Radix seu Folium Polygalae Fallacis) were used to reinforce the deficiency of the dragon and fire channels; Wujiapi (Cortex Acanthopanacis), Shengjiang (Rhizoma Zingiberis Recens), Xiangmao (Herba Cymbopogonis Citrari) and Aiye (Folium Artemisiae Argyi) were used to dispel wind and remove dampness; Gangbangui (Herba Polygoni Perfoliati) can promote diuresis; Lubianju (Herba Kalimeridis Indicae) were used to clear away heat. The orifices of the skin are important to the regulation of the qi and water passages because the decoction is absorbed through the skin to the dragon and fire channels running through the whole body. Then, the decoction and fluid exchange in the qi and water passages, resulting in acceleration of qi and blood circulation. This will make qi movement smooth. All the herbal medicinals combined can have a synergistic effect to purge excessive heat, tonify qi and blood, and regulate yin and yang, leading to good sleep at night.

（二）能啥累（湿疹）

2　Eczema ("Nenghanlei" in ZM)

1. 疾病概述

2.1　General description

能啥累指皮损呈多种形态，发无定位，易于湿烂渗液的一种瘙痒性、渗出性皮肤病证，是一种常见的过敏性炎症性皮肤病，相当于中医的湿疮和西医的湿疹。其特点为多形性皮疹，倾向湿润，对称分布，患者自觉剧烈瘙痒，易于反复发作。好发于面部、肘窝、腋窝、四肢屈侧及躯干等处。临床上一般分为急性湿疹（包括急性、亚急性和慢性湿疹急性发作 3 种）和慢性湿疹两大类，且二者又多相互转化。本病男女老少均可发生，无明显季节性。

"Nenghanlei", also known as "Shichuang" in TCM and eczema in WM, is a common allergic inflammatory skin disease characterized by variable forms of skin lesion, exudation and intense pruritus, liability to oozing, symmetrical distribution and repeated attack. It can occur all over the body, but is most common on the face, the insides of the elbows, the backs of the knees, flexural surfaces of the extremities and torso. From a clinical perspective, there are acute eczema (three stages of development: acute, subacute, and chronic) and chronic eczema, which can be turned into each other. The disease can occur at any age and in any season.

2. 病因病机

2.2　Cause and mechanism of disease

本病的发生主要与内部因素如精神情绪紧张、胃肠道刺激和外因如环境气候改变、接触过敏性物质或刺激性物质等原因有关。壮医认为，本病主要为湿热毒邪蕴阻龙路、火路或挟风邪、厉风、湿热客于肌肤所致；或因血虚、风袭或湿毒内盛致肌肤失于濡养而发病。慢性湿疹多由急性湿疹失治迁延转化而成。

Eczema can be caused by internal factors, such as mental and emotional stress, gastrointestinal irritation, and external factors, including climate changes and exposure to allergic or irritating substances. From the perspective of ZM, one main cause of eczema is stagnation of dampness-heat on the body superficies, which occurs when the dragon and fire channels are blocked by dampness and heat, or when pathogenic wind attacks the skin. Another main cause is the inadequate nourishment of the skin caused by blood deficiency combined with wind invasion, or exuberance of internal dampness. Eczema will become chronic if effective treatment is not given in the acute stage of it.

3. 诊查要点

2.3　Essentials for diagnosis

（1）诊断依据。

(1) Diagnosis criteria.

① 主症：皮损呈多样性，奇痒难忍，局部有渗出液，常对称分布，以头、面、四肢远端、阴囊等处多见，可泛发全身。

① Main symptoms: Variable forms of skin lesions, intense itching, exudation on some areas, symmetrical distribution. It can occur all over the body, but is commonly on the head, face, distal limbs and scrotum.

② 兼症：患处潮红或有红斑、丘疹、水疱、糜烂、痂皮、抓痕。

② Concurrent symptoms: Redness on disease sites, erythema, papules, blisters, erosion, scarring and scratching.

③ 甲诊：指甲颜色鲜红或青紫，半月痕暴露过多。

③ Nail examination: Fingernails are bright red or bluish purple, with large fingernail lunulae.

④ 目诊：勒答白睛上脉络弯曲多，弯度大，而且集中，靠近瞳仁，脉络边界浸润混浊，模糊不清。

④ Eye examination: Many large-radius bends are on the blood vessels on the white of the eyes, many of which are twisted and close to the pupils. The edges of the vessels are infiltrated and blurry.

（2）病证鉴别。

(2) Symptom differentiation.

① 痂怀。痂怀是一种慢性鳞屑性皮肤病。最初为针头或米粒大的红色丘疹，表面有少量白色鳞屑；随后丘疹逐渐扩大并融合，成为指甲、钱币或手掌大的大小不等的斑块，表面的鳞屑逐渐增厚。好发部位为四肢、头皮、颈项部、

低部和躯干，多对称发生。壮医认为，本病初起多由风毒、热毒、湿毒等外邪侵袭，阻于皮肤，蕴结不散而发，或嗜食辛辣肥甘之品，损伤"咪隆"（脾）、"咪胴"（肾），热毒内生，蕴于血分，两路受阻，感邪而发。本病迁延日久多耗伤气血，阴血亏虚，生风化燥，或病程日久，气滞血瘀，肌肤失养亦能发病。能唅累皮损呈多样性，局部有渗出液，常对称分布。

① Neurodermatitis ("Jiahuai" in ZM): A chronic scaly skin disease beginning with pinhead sized or rice sized red papules of which the surface is covered with a small amount of white scales. Then, these papules enlarge and coalesce into patches of varying sizes, such as the size of the nail, coin or hand palm, and at the same time, the layer of white scales becomes thicker. Neurodermatitis often symmetrically occurs on the extremities, scalp, nape and lower body. From the perspective of ZM, one main cause of neurodermatitis is the retention of wind, heat and dampness on the skin. Another cause is that pathogenic qi invades the two blocked channels. Eating spicy, greasy or sweet foods damages the spleen ("Milong" in the Zhuang language) and kidney ("Midong" in the Zhuang language), resulting in production of heat. Subsequently, the heat stagnates in the blood aspect and thus leads to the blockage of the channels. Long-term neurodermatitis makes qi and blood be consumed excessively, resulting in the deficiency of yin and blood. This will cause wind and dryness to be generated. Also, it will lead to qi stagnation and blood stasis, resulting in the inadequate nourishment of the skin. Consequently, neurodermatitis occurs. Eczema is characterized by variable forms of skin lesion, exudation in some areas and symmetrical distribution.

② 痤疮。痤疮是一种发于毛囊与皮脂腺的慢性炎症性皮肤病，因其初起损害多有粉刺，故又称粉刺。常好发于青春期男女。其临床主要表现为颜面、胸、背等处出现粟粒样丘疹如刺，有些融合成片，红肿或者有脓头，可挤出白色或黄白色碎米样粉汁，伴有轻微瘙痒或疼痛。痤疮的病程往往较长，常此起彼伏，部分青春期后可逐渐痊愈，但一些患者由于治疗不当或不注意卫生，可致其发为暗疮。壮医认为，痤疮多为素体阳盛，肺部蕴热，复感风湿热毒之邪熏蒸面部或脾胃湿热上蒸颜面，湿热瘀痰凝滞肌肤致三道两路受阻而发病。能唅累皮损呈多样性，奇痒难忍。

② Acne: A chronic inflammatory skin disease involving the hair follicles and sebaceous glands. Also known as pimple. This condition usually begins with the appearance of pimple-like bumps on the skin. It commonly occurs during puberty. The clinical manifestations include millet-like papules, cysts and nodules on the face, chest and back, some of them are in clusters. Normally, they are red and swollen, or filled with pus. The papules may cause slight itching or pain. When their walls break down, the white or yellowish sticky fluid will be discharged. Acne tends to run a long course because it waxes and wanes. Some patients can experience gradual recovery after puberty, but due to improper treatment or lack of hygiene, it will become lifelong acne. From the perspective of ZM, acne often occurs in people who are born with exuberant yang qi. Heat tends to stagnate in such people's lung. When the heat is combined with external wind, dampness or heat, or with dampness-heat in the spleen or stomach, the heat is more likely to rush onto the face. As a result, dampness-heat, blood stasis and phlegm stagnate on the body superficies, leading to the blockage of the three passages and two channels. Ultimately, acne occurs. Eczema is characterized by variable forms of skin lesion and intense pruritus.

4. 辨证论治

2.4　Syndrome differentiation and treatment

（1）治疗原则：祛风除湿，清热止痒，养血润燥。

(1) Treatment principles: Dispel wind, remove dampness, clear away heat, relieve itching, nourish blood and moisten dryness.

（2）证治分类。

(2) Classification of syndrome identification and treatment.

① 阳证：发病急，皮损潮红灼热，瘙痒无休，渗液流汁；伴身热、心烦口渴，大便干，尿短赤；舌质红，苔薄白或黄，脉大、急、有力。

① Yang syndrome: Abrupt onset, red skin lesions with a sensation of burning, persistent pruritus, exudation, generalized fever, vexation, thirst, dry stool, scanty dark urine, red tongue with white, thin or yellow coating, and large, rapid and forceful pulse.

治疗原则：祛风毒，除湿毒，清热毒，止痒。

Treatment principles: Dispel wind, remove dampness, clear away heat, and relieve itching.

选药：虎杖、海桐皮、白鲜皮、土荆皮、三叉苦、火炭母、杠板归、木蝴蝶。如湿毒重，可选用苦参、苍术、绵萆薢；如热毒重，可选用金银花、生石膏、野菊花、牡丹皮；如风毒重，可选用两面针、十大功劳；如瘙痒明显，可选用蛇床子、地肤子、火殃簕。

Prescription: Huzhang (Rhizoma et Radix Polygoni Cuspidati), Haitongpi (Cortex Erythrinae seu Kalopanacis), Baixianpi (Cortex Dictamni), Tujingpi (Cortex Pseudolaricis), Sanchaku (Folium et Ramulus Evodiae Leptae), Huotanmu (Herba Polygoni Chinensis), Gangbangui (Herba Polygoni Perfoliati) and Muhudie (Semen Oroxyli). For those with extreme dampness, add Kushen (Radix Sophorae Flavescentis), Cangzhu (Rhizoma Atractylodis), Mianbixie (Rhizoma Dioscoreae Septemlobae); for those with extreme heat, add Jinyinhua (Flos Lonicerae), Shengshigao (Gypsum Fibrosum), Yejuhua (Flos Chrysanthemi Indici) and Mudanpi (Cortex Moutan); for those with extreme wind, add Liangmianzhen (Radix Zanthoxyli) and Shidagonglao (Folium Mahoniae); for those with extreme intense pruritus, add Shechuangzi (Fructus Cnidii), Difuzi (Fructus Kochiae Scopariae) and Huoyangle (Folium Euphorbiae Antiquori).

② 阴证：发病较缓，皮损潮红，瘙痒，抓后糜烂渗液，可见鳞屑；伴有纳少，神疲，腹胀便溏；舌质淡胖或暗，苔白，脉小、有力。

② Yin syndrome: Slow onset, red skin lesions, erosion, exudation due to scratching, scaling, reduced appetite, lassitude, abdomen distension, loose stool; pale, plump or dark red tongue with white coating, thready and forceful pulse.

治疗原则：除湿毒，理气血，止痒。

Treatment principles: Remove dampness, regulate qi and blood, and relieve itching.

选药：三叉苦、败酱草、杠板归，半边莲，白鲜皮、百部、蛇床子。如寒毒明显，可选用桂枝、麻黄；如血瘀明显，可选用马鞭草、地骨皮；如脱屑明显，可选用当归、木鳖子；如瘙痒明显，可选用千里光、大叶桉。

Prescription: Sanchaku (Folium et Ramulus Evodiae Leptae), Baijiangcao

(Herba Patriniae), Gangbangui (Herba Polygoni Perfoliati), Banbianlian (Herba Lobeliae Chinensis), Baixianpi (Cortex Dictamni), Baibu (Radix Stemonae) and Shechuangzi (Fructus Cnidii). For those with obvious cold, add Guizhi (Ramulus Cinnamomi) and Mahuang (Herba Ephedrae); for those with obvious blood stasis, add Mabiancao (Herba Verbenae) and Digupi (Cortex Lycii); for those with obvious desquamation, add Danggui (Radix Angelicae Sinensis) and Mubiezi (Semen Momordicae); for those with obvious intense pruritus, add Qianliguang (Herba Senecionis Scandentis) and Daye'an (Folium Eucalypti Robustae).

③虚证：患病日久，皮损色暗或色素沉着，剧痒，或皮损粗糙肥厚；伴口干不欲饮，纳差腹胀；舌淡，苔白，脉小、无力。

③ Deficiency syndrome: Long-term course, dark brown skin lesions, or with pigmentation, intense itching, or thickened skin lesions, a sensation of dryness in the mouth without desire to drink, reduced appetite, abdomen distension, pale tongue with white coating, thready and weak pulse.

治疗原则：补虚祛毒，理气血，润燥止痒。

Treatment principles: Reinforce deficiency, remove toxins, regulate qi and blood, moisten dryness and relieve itching.

选药：白鲜皮、当归、蒸黄精、杠板归、海桐皮、救必应、蒲公英、土茯苓。

Prescription: Baixianpi (Cortex Dictamni), Danggui (Radix Angelicae Sinensis), steamed Huangjing (Rhizoma Polygonati), Gangbangui (Herba Polygoni Perfoliati), Haitongpi (Cortex Erythrinae seu Kalopanacis), Jiubiying (Cortex Ilicis Rotundae), Pugongying (Herba Taraxaci) and Tufuling (Rhizoma Smilacis Glabrae).

如虚证明显，可选用黄花倒水莲、鸡血藤、千斤拔；如寒证明显，可选用麻黄、桂枝；如皮损粗糙肥厚明显，可选用虎杖、牡丹皮、土大黄；如瘙痒明显，可选用黄柏、马齿苋、浮萍。

For those with severe deficiency syndrome, add Huanghuadaoshuilian (Radix seu Folium Polygalae Fallacis), Jixueteng (Caulis Spatholobi), Qianjinba (Radix et Caulis Flemingiae); for those with obvious cold, add Mahuang (Herba Ephedrae) and Guizhi (Ramulus Cinnamomi); for those with obvious thickened skin lesion, add Huzhang (Rhizoma et Radix Polygoni Cuspidati), Mudanpi (Cortex Moutan) and

Tudahuang (Radix Rumicis Obtusifolii); for those with obvious intense puritus, add Huangbo (Cortex Phellodendri Chinensis), Machixian (Herba Portulacae) and Fuping (Herba Spirodelae).

5. 预防调护

2.5　Prevention and care

过敏性体质或有过敏性家族史者，要避免各种外界刺激，如热水烫洗、搔抓、日晒等，尽量避免食用易致敏和刺激性的食物。生活要规律，注意劳逸结合。衣着宜宽松，以减少摩擦刺激，勿使化纤品及毛织品直接接触皮肤。

People with allergic constitution or family history of allergies should avoid external stimuli, such as bathing with hot water, scratching and sun exposure, as well as allergenic and stimulating foods. They should have a regular life, maintain a work-life balance and wear loose clothing to reduce irritation caused by friction. Clothing made of chemical fibers and wool should not directly contact the skin.

6. 医案选读

2.6　Selected case readings

【病案一】

［Case 1］

龙某，男，40 岁，2019 年 6 月 20 日初诊。

Patient: Long, a 40-year-old man, his first visit was on June 20, 2019.

主诉：反复皮肤瘙痒 6 个月。

Chief complaint:"I have had recurrent skin pruritus for six months."

现病史：2019 年 1 月无明显诱因下出现全身丘疹（图 25），高于皮面，边界清楚，伴皮肤瘙痒，曾到医院就诊，给予中药内服，效果欠佳。舌红，苔薄黄，脉浮。

History of present illness: Papules occurred all over the patient's body in January 2019 without any apparent reasons (Fig. 25). These papules were elevated, demarcated and pruritic. He was treated with oral administration of traditional Chinese medicine at our hospital but the efficacy was not good. His tongue is red with yellow, thin coating. His pulse is floating.

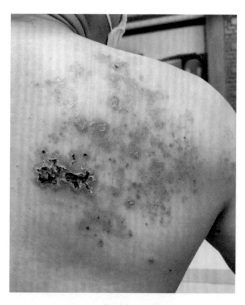

图 25 能啥累（阳证）
Fig. 25 "Nenghanlei" (yang syndrome)

目诊：白睛脉络色红，迂曲。甲诊：甲色偏红。壮医诊断：能啥累（阳证）。中医诊断：湿疮。西医诊断：湿疹。

Eye examination: The blood vessels on the white of the eyes are red and curved.

Nail examination: The nails are reddish.

Diagnosis in ZM: "Nenghanlei" characterized by yang syndrome.

Diagnosis in TCM: Eczema.

Diagnosis in WM: Eczema.

治疗原则：祛风除湿，清热止痒。

Treatment principles: Dispel wind, remove dampness, clear away heat and relieve itching.

治疗：壮医药浴疗法。

Treatment method: The ZM medicated bath therapy.

处方：虎杖 50 g，海桐皮 50 g，白鲜皮 50 g，土荆皮 10 g，三叉苦 50 g，火炭母 50 g，绵萆薢 50 g，杠板归 50 g，地肤子 20 g，苦参 30 g，木蝴蝶 30 g，牡丹皮 30 g。

Prescription: Huzhang (Rhizoma et Radix Polygoni Cuspidati) 50 g, Haitongpi

(Cortex Erythrinae seu Kalopanacis) 50 g, Baixianpi (Cortex Dictamni) 50 g, Tujingpi (Cortex Pseudolaricis) 10 g, Sanchaku (Folium et Ramulus Evodiae Leptae) 50 g, Huotanmu (Herba Polygoni Chinensis) 50 g, Mianbixie (Rhizoma Dioscoreae Septemlobae) 50 g, Gangbangui (Herba Polygoni Perfoliati) 50 g, Difuzi (Fructus Kochiae Scopariae) 20 g, Kushen (Radix Sophorae Flavescentis) 30 g, Muhudie (Semen Oroxyli) 30 g and Mudanpi (Cortex Moutan) 30 g.

二诊（2019 年 7 月 2 日）：经壮医药浴疗法治疗 5 次后，皮疹明显缓解。

Second visit (on July 2, 2019): After taking the ZM medicated bath for five times, many of the papules had vanished.

按语：本案患者出现湿疹，舌红，苔薄黄，脉浮，属阳证。乃湿热毒邪挟风邪蕴阻龙路、火路，客于肌肤所致。治宜以祛风除湿、清热止痒为主。采用壮医药浴疗法治疗，方中使用海桐皮、白鲜皮、绵萆薢、土荆皮祛风除湿，虎杖、火炭母、地肤子、三叉苦、苦参清热止痒，杠板归加强除湿毒，木蝴蝶、牡丹皮加强清热毒。诸药合用，除肌肤风毒、湿毒、热毒，通畅龙路、火路，皮疹、瘙痒自除。

Summary statement: The eczema the patient had and his red tongue with yellow, thin coating and floating pulse signified yang syndrome. Dampness-heat combined with pathogenic wind blocked the dragon and fire channels and, subsequently, stagnated on the body superficies. This led to appearance of eczema. Therefore, it was applicable to dispel wind, remove dampness, clear away heat and relieve itching. In terms of the herbal medicinals used in the ZM medicated bath therapy, Haitongpi (Cortex Erythrinae seu Kalopanacis), Baixianpi (Cortex Dictamni), Mianbixie (Rhizoma Dioscoreae Septemlobae) and Tujingpi (Cortex Pseudolaricis) were used to dispel wind and remove dampness; Huzhang (Rhizoma et Radix Polygoni Cuspidati), Huotanmu (Herba Polygoni Chinensis), Difuzi (Fructus Kochiae Scopariae), Sanchaku (Folium et Ramulus Evodiae Leptae) and Kushen (Radix Sophorae Flavescentis) were used to clear away heat and relieve itching; Gangbangui (Herba Polygoni Perfoliati) can remove dampness toxin; Muhudie (Semen Oroxyli) and Mudanpi (Cortex Moutan) were used to clear away heat. All the herbal medicinals combined took the synergistic effect to dispel wind, remove dampness and clear away heat stagnating on the body superficies to unblock the dragon and fire channels. Consequently, eczema and itching vanish.

【病案二】

［Case 2］

唐某，女，33 岁，2020 年 9 月 3 日初诊。

Patient: Tang, a 33-year-old woman, her first visit was on September 3, 2020.

主诉：反复脚部湿疹 6 年。

Chief complaint:"I have had eczema on my feet for 6 years."

现病史：6 年前无明显诱因下出现脚部湿疹（图 26），有渗液，瘙痒明显，经治疗可缓解，但易反复发作，伴下肢怕冷，纳可，小便调。舌暗红，舌尖红，苔白腻，脉滑。

History of present illness: Eczema appeared on the feet without any apparent reasons six years ago (Fig. 26). It was manifested by exudation and intense pruritus. The symptoms could be relieved after treatment but reappeared. She reported intolerance of cold in her lower limbs, good appetite and normal urination frequency. Her tongue is dark red with red tongue-tip and white, greasy coating. Her pulse is slippery.

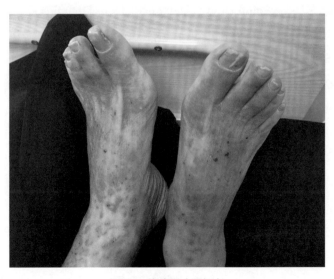

图 26　能唅累（阴证）
Fig. 26 "Nenghanlei" (yin syndrome)

目诊：白睛脉络色淡，迂曲。甲诊：甲色偏淡。壮医诊断：能啥累（阴证）。中医诊断：湿疮。西医诊断：慢性湿疹。

Eye examination: The blood vessels on the white of the eyes are reddish and curved.

Nail examination: The nails are pale.

Diagnosis in ZM:"Nenghanlei" characterized by yin syndrome.

Diagnosis in TCM: Eczema.

Diagnosis in WM: Eczema.

治疗原则：祛风除湿，散寒养血。

Treatment principles: Dispel wind, remove dampness, dissipate cold and nourish blood.

治疗：壮医药浴疗法。

Treatment method: The ZM medicated bath therapy.

处方：三叉苦 30 g，蛇床子 15 g，百部 15 g，地骨皮 15 g，杠板归 30 g，半边莲 30 g，马鞭草 30 g，桂枝 20 g，麻黄 20 g，白鲜皮 30 g，当归 10 g，败酱草 20 g，千里光 20 g。

Prescription: Sanchaku (Folium et Ramulus Evodiae Leptae) 30 g, Shechuangzi (Fructus Cnidii) 15 g, Baibu (Radix Stemonae) 15 g, Digupi (Cortex Lycii) 15 g, Gangbangui (Herba Polygoni Perfoliati) 30 g, Banbianlian (Herba Lobeliae Chinensis) 30 g, Mabiancao (Herba Verbenae) 30 g, Guizhi (Ramulus Cinnamomi) 20 g, Mahuang (Herba Ephedrae) 20 g, Baixianpi (Cortex Dictamni) 30 g, Danggui (Radix Angelicae Sinensis) 10 g, Baijiangcao (Herba Patriniae) 20 g, Qianliguang (Herba Senecionis Scandentis) 20 g.

二诊（2020 年 7 月 16 日）：经壮医药浴疗法治疗 7 次，皮疹明显缓解。

Second visit (on July 16, 2020): After the patient took the ZM medicated bath seven times, many of the rashes vanished.

按语：本案患者出现反复湿疹发作，伴怕冷现象，舌暗红，舌尖红，苔白腻，脉滑，属湿毒之阴证。乃湿毒内盛所致肌肤失于濡养而发病。治宜以祛风除湿、散寒养血为主。采用壮医药浴疗法治疗，方中使用蛇床子、白鲜皮、马鞭草祛风除湿，湿毒郁久易化热故使用三叉苦、半边莲、地骨皮辅以清热毒，杠板归利水道及加强除湿毒，麻黄、桂枝散寒毒，当归养血，百部、千里光止痒，败酱草化瘀毒。诸药合用，共奏祛风除湿、散寒养血之功，肌肤濡润如常，皮疹、瘙痒自除。

Summary statement: Eczema on the patient's feet waxed and waned for six years. She reported intolerance of cold. Her tongue was dark red with red tongue-tip and white, greasy coating. Her pulse was slippery. These manifestations signified yin syndrome of dampness. Exuberance of interior dampness caused the inadequate nourishment of the skin, resulting in appearance of eczema. Therefore, it was applicable to dispel wind, remove dampness, dissipate cold and nourish blood. In terms of the herbal medicinals used in the ZM medicated bath therapy, Shechuangzi (Fructus Cnidii), Baixianpi (Cortex Dictamni) and Mabiancao (Herba Verbenae) were used to dispel wind and remove dampness; since long-term retention of dampness tends to transform into heat, Sanchaku (Folium et Ramulus Evodiae Leptae), Banbianlian (Herba Lobeliae Chinensis) and Digupi (Cortex Lycii) were used to clear away heat; Gangbangui (Herba Polygoni Perfoliati) is excellent at inducing diuresis, so it was used to assist in removing dampness; Mahuang (Herba Ephedrae) and Guizhi (Ramulus Cinnamomi) were used to dissipate cold; Danggui (Radix Angelicae Sinensis) was used to nourish blood; Baibu (Radix Stemonae) and Qianliguang (Herba Senecionis Scandentis) were used to relieve itching; and Baijiangcao (Herba Patriniae) was used to resolve blood stasis. All the herbal medicinals combined took the synergistic effect to dispel wind, remove dampness, dissipate cold and nourish blood. Consequently, dry skin was moistened, and eczema and itching vanished.

【病案三】

［Case 3］

林某，女，39 岁，2020 年 6 月 9 日初诊。

Patient: Lin, a 39-year-old woman, her first visit was on June 9, 2020.

主诉：双手皮疹 1 年。

Chief complaint:"I have had eczema on my hands for one year."

现病史：患者述 1 年前出现双手皮疹（图 27），瘙痒明显，治疗后未见明显效果。刻下见双手手掌面皮肤变厚、角化，瘙痒明显，纳少，寐可。舌淡，苔白，脉细滑。

History of present illness: Eczema appeared on the patient's hands one year ago (Fig. 27). It was manifested by intense pruritus. The symptoms were not relieved after treatment.

Current symptoms: Thickened palmar skin, intense pruritus, reduced appetite, restful sleep, pale tongue with white coating and thready, slippery pulse.

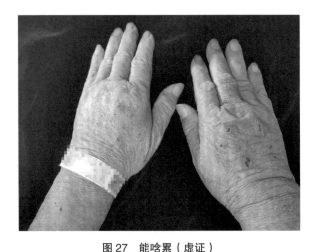

图 27　能唅累（虚证）
Fig. 27 "Nenghanlei" (deficiency syndrome)

目诊：白睛脉络色淡。甲诊：甲色偏淡。壮医诊断：能唅累（虚证）。中医诊断：湿疮。西医诊断：慢性湿疹。

Eye examination: The blood vessels on the white of the eyes are reddish.

Nail examination: The nails are pale.

Diagnosis in ZM:"Nenghanlei" characterized by deficiency syndrome.

Diagnosis in TCM: Eczema.

Diagnosis in WM: Chronic eczema.

治疗原则：补虚祛毒，理气血，润燥止痒。

Treatment principles: Reinforce deficiency, remove toxins, regulate qi and blood, moisten dryness and relieve itching.

治疗：壮医药浴疗法。

Treatment method: The ZM medicated bath therapy.

处方：白鲜皮 30 g，当归 10 g，蒸黄精 15 g，杠板归 30 g，海桐皮 30 g，虎杖 30 g，黄柏 30 g，救必应 30 g，桂枝 20 g，麻黄 20 g，马齿苋 15 g，蒲公英 30 g，土茯苓 30 g，黄花倒水莲 30 g。

Prescription: Baixianpi (Cortex Dictamni) 30 g, Danggui (Radix Angelicae Sinensis) 10 g, steamed Huangjing (Rhizonma Polygonati) 15 g, Gangbangui (Herba Polygoni Perfoliati) 30 g, Haitongpi (Cortex Erythrinae seu Kalopanacis) 30 g, Huzhang (Rhizoma et Radix Polygoni Cuspidati) 30 g, Huangbo (Cortex Phellodendri Chinensis) 30 g, Jiubiying (Cortex Ilicis Rotundae) 30 g, Guizhi (Ramulus Cinnamomi) 20 g, Mahuang (Herba Ephedrae) 20 g, Machixian (Herba Portulacae) 15 g, Pugongying (Herba Taraxaci) 30 g, Tufuling (Rhizoma Smilacis Glabrae) 30 g, Huanghuadaoshuilian (Radix seu Folium Polygalae Fallacis) 30 g.

二诊（2020 年 7 月 16 日）：经壮医药浴疗法治疗 10 次后，皮肤变厚感减轻，瘙痒明显缓解。

Second visit (on July 16, 2020): After the patient took the ZM medicated bath ten times, skin thickening had been reduced and pruritus had been significantly relieved.

按语：本案患者 1 年前出现双手手掌面皮肤变厚、角化，瘙痒明显，舌淡，苔白，脉细滑，属虚证。治宜以补虚祛毒、理气血、润燥止痒为主。采用壮医药浴疗法治疗，方中使用黄花倒水莲、当归、蒸黄精补虚养血润燥，白鲜皮、海桐皮祛风除湿，杠板归、马齿苋、救必应、土茯苓加强除湿毒。寒毒内阻使皮肤变厚、角化，故用桂枝、麻黄散寒毒，湿毒郁久化热致瘙痒明显；故用虎杖、黄柏、蒲公英辅以清热毒。诸药合用，共奏补虚祛毒、理气血、润燥止痒之功，瘙痒自除。

Summary statement: One year ago, the patient's palmar skin became thickened, accompanied by intense pruritus. Her tongue was pale with white coating. Her pulse was thready and slippery. These manifestations signified deficiency syndrome. Therefore, it was applicable to reinforce deficiency, remove toxins, regulate qi and blood, moisten dryness and relieve itching. In terms of the herbal medicinals used in the ZM medicated bath therapy, Huanghuadaoshuilian (Radix seu Folium Polygalae Fallacis), Danggui (Radix Angelicae Sinensis) and steamed Huangjing (Rhizoma

Polygonati) were used to reinforce deficiency, nourish blood and moisten dryness; Baixianpi (Cortex Dictamni) and Haitongpi (Cortex Erythrinae seu Kalopanacis) were used to dispel wind and remove dampness; Gangbangui (Herba Polygoni Perfoliati), Machixian (Herba Portulacae), Jiubiying (Cortex Ilicis Rotundae) and Tufuling (Rhizoma Smilacis Glabrae) were used to remove dampness; since the skin was thickened due to cold, Guizhi (Ramulus Cinnamomi) and Mahuang (Herba Ephedrae) were used to dissipate cold; since transformation into heat due to long-term retention of dampness led to intense pruritus, Huzhang (Rhizoma et Radix Polygoni Cuspidati), Huangbo (Cortex Phellodendri Chinensis) and Pugongying (Herba Taraxaci) were used to clear away heat. All the herbal medicinals combined took the synergistic effect to reinforce deficiency, remove toxins, regulate qi and blood, moisten dryness and relieve itching. Finally, pruritus vanished.

（三）乒产呱（产后病）

3　Postpartum diseases ("Pingchangua" in ZM)

1. 疾病概述

3.1　General description

产妇在产褥期内发生的与分娩或产褥有关的疾病称为乒产呱。产妇分娩耗伤气血，产褥期妇女处于"多虚多瘀"的状态之中，又有哺育婴儿之劳顿，所以"致疾之易，而去疾之患，莫甚于此"。因此，必须加强产褥期疾病预防与保健，以利于母婴健康。

"Pingchangua" refers to diseases occurring in the puerperal period, related to labor and puerperium. Depletion of qi and blood in childbirth makes women in the postpartum period have qi deficiency and blood stasis. Besides, they are exhausted due to breastfeeding. As a result, they are highly likely to get sick, but it is difficult for them to recover. Therefore, it is necessary to improve postpartum care to strengthen maternal and infant health.

本病相当于中医的产后病，西医的产褥期疾病亦可参考本病进行诊治。

"Pingchangua" is the same as puerperal diseases in TCM and postpartum diseases in WM, so the treatment of these medical conditions can refer to that of

"Pingchangua".

2. 病因病机

3.2　Cause and mechanism of disease

（1）产后津血损伤。临产时用力及产伤出血，使阴勒（血）流失，津液耗损。

(1) Loss of fluid-blood after childbirth. Bleeding during and after childbirth leads to excessive consumption of blood ("Le" in the Zhuang language) and body fluid.

（2）瘀血内阻。产时耗气伤血，脉络空虚，在复原过程中，瘀血易停、滞留。

(2) Internal retention of blood stasis. Excessive consumption of qi and blood during delivery leads to meridian emptiness. During recovery, static blood tends to stagnate.

（3）毒气内侵或饮食房劳所伤。产后龙路空虚，起居不慎，邪毒乘虚而入；产后元气、津血俱伤，生活稍有不慎或调摄失当，为饮食、房劳所伤，可使"嘘"（气）、"勒"（血）及内脏功能失常而变生诸疾。

(3) Invasion of pathogenic qi or internal injury due to improper diet or excessive sexual consumption. Pathogenic qi attacks the weak body which is caused by the emptiness of the dragon channel and irregular life schedule after childbirth. The original qi, body fluid and blood are excessively consumed after childbirth. Under such circumstances, irregular life schedule, improper diet or excessive sexual activity will make qi ("Xu" in the Zhuang language) and blood ("Le" in the Zhuang language) in zang-fu organs insufficient, leading to the dysfunction of these organs. Consequently, diseases occur.

3. 诊查要点

3.3　Essentials for diagnosis

（1）诊断依据。

3.3.1　Diagnosis criteria

① 主症：产后少气懒言，神疲乏力，形体消瘦，声低息微，活动时诸症加重，容易伤风感冒。

① Main symptoms: Shortness of breath, no desire to speak, lassitude, weak constitution, low voice with feeble breathing, which are aggravated by exertion, and liability to common cold.

② 兼症：发热自汗，心悸失眠，心烦易怒，不思饮食，大便不调，视物不清，头晕眼花，耳鸣，腰膝酸软。

② Concurrent symptoms: Generalized fever, spontaneous sweating, palpitation, sleeplessness, vexation, irritability, reduced appetite, irregular bowel movements, blurred vision, dizziness, tinnitus, soreness and weakness in the lower back and knees.

③ 甲诊：指甲颜色苍白或淡白，半月痕暴露过多，按压甲尖后放开，指甲颜色不恢复或久久未恢复原色，可见葱管甲、竹笋甲、横沟甲、白色甲或萎缩甲。

③ Nail examination: Fingernails are pale or slightly pale with large fingernail lunulae. When a fingernail stops being pressed, the color of the fingernail will not return or return slowly. There are Beau's lines on the nail bed, the nail looks like bamboo shoot or scallion, or the nails are atrophied, which may be accompanied by partial or entire white nail bed.

④ 目诊：勒答白睛上脉络弯曲多，弯度大，脉络多而集中，靠近瞳仁，可有瘀点。

④ Eye examination: Many large-radius bends are on the blood vessels on the white of the eyes, many of which are visible, twisted and close to the pupils, or with petechiae.

（2）病证鉴别。

3.3.2　Symptom differentiation

① 钵痨。钵痨为正气不足，结核杆菌侵袭所致；病位主要在气道；具有传染性；临床主要表现出咳嗽、咯血、潮热、盗汗、消瘦等症状。钵痨亦可由肺病波及他脏，发生气阴亏耗或阴损及阳、阴阳两虚的病变。乒产呱涉及多个脏腑，以咪花肠（胞宫）、脾肾为主；无传染性；产后多虚多瘀为其基本病机；临床表现为脏腑气血阴阳亏虚的多种证候。

① Lung phthisis ("Bolao" in ZM): A infectious disease caused by invasion of Mycobacterium tuberculosis (MTB) bacteria when healthy qi is insufficient. The disease site is in the qi passage. The main clinical manifestations include cough, hemoptysis, tidal fever, night sweats and marasmus. Lung phthisis affects the lungs and may spread to other organs. It can lead to excessive consumption of yin and qi. It can also cause yin impairment to affect yang, resulting in dual deficiency of yin and yang. In contrast, postpartum diseases ("Pingchangua" in ZM) involve many organs, but often affect the womb ("Mihuachang" in the Zhuang language), spleen and kidney. These diseases are not contagious. Their basic pathogenesis is deficiency and blood stasis. Their clinical manifestations are variable signs of the deficiency qi, blood, yin and yang in zang-fu organs.

② 更年期综合征。更年期综合征为妇女于 45 ～ 55 岁由于卵巢功能退行性改变，月经逐渐停止来潮而进入绝经期所出现的一系列内分泌失调和自主神经功能紊乱症候。主要表现为经行紊乱，面部潮红，易出汗，烦躁易怒，精神疲倦，头晕耳鸣，心悸失眠，甚至情志异常；有的还伴有尿频、尿急、食欲不振等，可持续 2 ～ 3 年之久。壮医认为，本病乃肾阴不足，阳失潜藏或肾阳虚衰所致。而乒产呱为产后引起，有明确的发病时期。

② Climacteric syndrome: A disorder normally occurring in women between the ages of 45 and 55. Due to degenerative changes in the ovary, menstruation becomes less frequent and eventually stops altogether. This causes endocrine disorders and autonomic dysfunction symptoms. The clinical manifestations include irregular periods, flushed face, liability to sweating, vexation, irritability, lassitude, dizziness, tinnitus, palpitation, insomnia and emotional disorders. Some women may experience frequent urination, urinary urgency and reduced appetite. The symptoms can last for two to three years. From the perspective of ZM, menopause is caused by kidney yin insufficiency, failure to subdue yang or debilitation of kidney yang. In contrast, postpartum diseases occur after childbirth with a clear onset.

4. 辨证论治

3.4 Syndrome differentiation and treatment

（1）治疗原则：扶正补虚，辅以祛毒。

(1) Treatment principles: Reinforce the healthy qi and reinforce deficiency with due consideration to toxin removal.

（2）证治分类。

(2) Classification of syndrome identification and treatment.

① 阳证：头晕耳鸣，口眼干涩，心烦失眠，潮热盗汗，勒答脉络粗大，色深红或红紫，曲张明显。

① Yang syndrome: Dizziness, tinnitus, bitter and dry mouth, dry and uncomfortable eyes, vexation, insomnia, tidal fever, night sweats, dark red or reddish violet blood vessels of the eyes, which are obviously enlarged and twisted.

治疗原则：滋阴补虚，畅气郁，清热毒。

Treatment principles: Replenish yin, reinforce deficiency, relieve qi depression and clear away heat.

选药：牛大力、扶芳藤、鸡血藤、香茅、艾叶、生姜。

Prescription: Niudali (Radix Millettiae Speciosae), Fufangteng (Caulis Euonymi Fortunei cum Foliis), Jixueteng (Caulis Spatholobi), Xiangmao (Herba Cymbopogonis Citrari), Aiye (Folium Artemisiae Argyi) and Shengjiang (Rhizoma Zingiberis Recens).

如虚证明显，可选用当归藤、杜仲藤；如瘀毒明显，可选用千斤拔、五加皮、鹰不扑；如气郁明显，可选用郁金、姜黄、莪术；如热毒明显，可选用葫芦茶、木贼；如湿毒明显，可选用黄柏、苍术。

For those with obvious deficiency syndrome, add Dangguiteng (*Embelia Parviflora* Wall.) and Duzhongteng (Cortex Parabarii); for those with obvious blood stasis, add Qianjinba (Radix et Caulis Flemingiae), Wujiapi (Cortex Acanthopanacis) and Yingbupu (Radix Araliae Armatae); for those with obvious qi depression, add Yujin (Radix Curumae), Jianghuang (Rhizoma Curcumae Longae) and Ezhu (Rhizoma Curcumae); for those with obvious heat, add Hulucha (Herba Tadehagi Triquetri) and Muzei (Herba Equiseti Hiemalis); for those with obvious dampness, add Huangbo (Cortex Phellodendri Chinensis) and Cangzhu (Rhizoma Atractylodis).

② 阴证：形寒肢冷，短气自汗，心悸气喘，身疲乏力，面色苍白，勒答脉络色淡、弯曲、边界混浊／散乱、模糊不清，末端有瘀点；上白睛有雾斑或瘀斑。

② Yin syndrome: Cold limbs, shortness of breath, spontaneous sweating, palpitation with feeble breathing, lassitude, pale complexion, reddish curved blood vessels of the eyes with indefinite or stretched border and petechiae on the ends, and cloudy or blood spots on the upper white of the eyes.

治疗原则：扶阳补虚，除瘀毒，祛风毒，散寒毒。

Treatment principles: Reinforce yang and deficiency, and remove blood stasis, dispel wind and dissipate cold.

选药：黄花倒水莲、牛大力、艾叶、路路通、走马胎、生姜。如虚证明显，可选用扶芳藤、五指毛桃；如瘀毒明显，可选用益母草、牛膝、鸡屎藤；如寒毒明显，可选用桂枝、威灵仙；如风毒明显，可选用苏木、防风、伸筋草、红花；如湿毒明显，可选用葛根、草豆蔻、厚朴。

Prescription: Huanghuadaoshuilian (Radix seu Folium Polygalae Fallacis), Niudali (Radix Millettiae Speciosae), Aiye (Folium Artemisiae Argyi), Lulutong (Fructus Liquidambaris), Zoumatai (Radix et Rhizoma Ardisiae Gigantifoliae) and Shengjiang (Rhizoma Zingiberis Recens). For those with obvious deficiency syndrome, add Fufangteng (Caulis Euonymi Fortunei cum Foliis) and Wuzhimaotao (Radix Fici Hirtae); for those with obvious blood stasis, add Yimucao (Herba Leonuri), Niuxi (Radix Achyranthis Bidentatae) and Jishiteng (Herba Paederiae); for those with obvious cold, add Guizhi (Ramulus Cinnamomi) and Weilingxian (Radix et Rhizoma Clematidis); for those with obvious wind, add Sumu (Lignum Sappan), Fangfeng (Radix Saposhnikoviae), Shenjincao (Herba Lycopodii) and Honghua (Flos Carthami); for those with obvious dampness, add Gegen (Radix Puerariae), Caodoukou (Semen Alpiniae Katsumadai) and Houpo (Cortex Magnoliae Officinalis).

5. 预防调护

3.5　Prevention and care

产后病患者由于正气不足，卫外不固，容易招致外邪入侵，应尽量少触外邪。饮食调理以富于营养、易于消化、不伤脾胃为宜。少食辛辣厚味、滋腻、生冷之物，戒除烟酒。生活起居规律，动静结合，劳逸适度，节制房事。保持情绪稳定，舒畅乐观，有利于产后病的康复。

A patient with a postpartum disease should avoid external pathogenic factors because the deficiency of healthy qi combined with insecurity of defense qi makes her body tend to be attacked by them. Foods she consumes should be nutritious, digestible and nice for the spleen and stomach rather than spicy, salty, greasy and uncooked. Smoking and alcohol consumption is forbidden. She should have a regular life schedule, with a proper balance between work and rest, and avoid excess of sexual activity. She should also maintain emotional stability and positive attitude because they are conducive to the recovery from diseases.

6. 医案选读

3.6　Selected case readings

【病案一】

［Case 1］

韦某，女，33 岁，2020 年 5 月 15 日初诊。

Patient: Wei, a 33-year-old woman, her first visit was on May 15, 2020.

主诉：产后腰痛、睡眠欠佳 1 月余。

Chief complaint:"I have had postpartum lumbago and restless sleep for more than one month."

现病史：1 个多月前产后开始出现腰痛、睡眠欠佳，纳一般，大便秘结。舌暗，苔黄腻（图 28）。脉弦。

History of present illness: The patient reported postpartum lumbago that occurred more than one month ago, restless sleep, reduced appetite and constipation. Her tongue is dark red with yellow, greasy coating (Fig. 28). Her pulse is wiry.

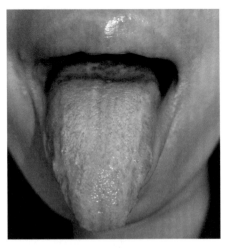

图 28　乒产呱（阳证）
Fig. 28　"Pingchangua"（yang syndrome）

目诊：勒答脉络粗大，色深红，曲张明显。甲诊：甲色偏红。壮医诊断：乒产呱（阳证）。中医诊断：产后病。西医诊断：产褥期疾病。

Eye examination: The blood vessels of the eyes are dark red, and apparently enlarged and twisted.

Nail examination: The nails are reddish.

Diagnosis in ZM:"Pingchangua" characterized by yang syndrome.

Diagnosis in TCM: Puerperal diseases.

Diagnosis in WM: Postpartum diseases.

治疗原则：补虚，畅气郁，清热毒。

Treatment principles: Reinforce deficiency, relieve qi depression and clear away heat.

治疗：壮医药浴疗法。

Treatment method: The ZM medicated bath therapy.

处方：牛大力 50 g，扶芳藤 30 g，鸡血藤 30 g，当归藤 30 g，杜仲藤 30 g，香茅 20 g，黄柏 20 g，艾叶 20 g，生姜 50 g。

Prescription: Niudali (Radix Millettiae Speciosae) 50 g, Fufangteng (Caulis Euonymi Fortunei cum Foliis) 30 g, Jixueteng (Caulis Spatholobi) 30 g, Dangguiteng (*Embelia Parviflora* Wall.) 30 g, Duzhongteng (Cortex Parabarii) 30 g, Xiangmao (Herba Cymbopogonis Citrari) 20 g, Huangbo (Cortex Phellodendri Chinensis) 20 g, Aiye (Folium Artemisiae Argyi) 20 g and Shengjiang (Rhizoma Zingiberis Recens) 50 g.

二诊（2020 年 5 月 22 日）：经壮医药浴疗法治疗 5 次，腰痛明显缓解，二便正常，睡眠、饮食较前改善，继予药浴 3 次，巩固疗效。

Second visit (on May 22, 2020): After the patient took the ZM medicated bath five times, postpartum lumbago had been relieved. She reported normal urination frequency, regular bowel movements, better sleep and appetite. Accordingly, she was instructed to take the ZM medicated bath for another three times to consolidate the efficacy.

按语：本案患者产褥期出现腰痛，睡眠欠佳，大便秘结，舌暗，苔黄腻，脉弦，属阳证。产后龙路空虚，起居不慎，邪毒乘虚而入；产后元气、津血俱伤，生活稍有不慎或调摄失当，为饮食、房劳所伤，可使"嘘"（气）、"勒"（血）及内脏功能失常而变生诸疾。腰痛、舌暗缘自龙路不通，瘀毒内阻，火路不通可致睡眠欠佳，谷道虚损不足、湿毒内生可致大便秘结，治宜以通调龙路、火路，补虚损，除瘀毒湿毒为主。采用壮医药浴疗法治疗，方中使用牛大力、扶芳藤、鸡血藤通调龙路火路，补虚损，当归藤、杜仲藤除瘀毒，强筋骨，香茅、艾叶、生姜散风毒，除湿毒，黄柏利湿热。诸药通过药浴合用，可使道路畅通，气血滋生，三气同步，腰痛、睡眠欠佳自除。

Summary statement: The patient reported postpartum lumbago, restless sleep, reduced appetite and constipation. Her tongue was dark red with yellow, greasy coating. Her pulse was wiry. These manifestations signified yang syndrome. Pathogenic factors invade the weak body which is caused by the emptiness of the dragon channel and irregular life schedule after childbirth. The original qi, body fluid and blood are excessively consumed during and after childbirth. Under such circumstances, irregular life schedule, improper diet and excess of sexual activity made qi ("Xu" in the Zhuang language) and blood ("Le" in the zhuang language) in zang-fu organs insufficient, leading to the dysfunction of these organs. Consequently, diseases occur. Postpartum lumbago and the dark red edge of the patient's tongue mean that the dragon channel was blocked and blood stasis stagnated in her body. The obstruction of the fire channel led to restless sleep. The consumption in the grain passage and internal dampness led to constipation. Therefore, it was applicable to regulate the dragon and fire channels, reduce consumption and remove blood stasis and dampness. In terms of the herbal medicinals used in the ZM medicated bath therapy, Niudali (Radix Millettiae Speciosae), Fufangteng (Caulis Euonymi Fortunei cum Foliis) and Jixueteng (Caulis Spatholobi) were used to regulate the dragon and fire channels and reduce consumption; Dangguiteng (*Embelia Parviflora* Wall.) and Duzhongteng (Cortex Parabarii) were used to remove blood stasis and strengthen tendons and bones; Xiangmao (Herba Cymbopogonis Citrari), Aiye (Folium Artemisiae Argyi) and Shengjiang (Rhizoma Zingiberis Recens) were used to dispel wind and remove dampness; and Huangbo (Cortex Phellodendri Chinensis) was used to induce dampness-heat. All the herbal medicinals combined took synergistic effect to unblock the two channels, nourish blood and qi and make the heaven-qi, earth-qi and human-qi synchronized. Consequently, the lumbago vanished and sleep quality was improved.

【病案二】

［Case 2］

孙某，女，33 岁，2020 年 12 月 1 日初诊。

Patient: Sun, a 33-year-old woman, her first visit was on December 1, 2020.

主诉：产后畏风 1 周。

Chief complaint:"I have had intolerance of wind for one week."

现病史：产后 31 天即 1 周前开始出现畏风，自觉身重乏力，纳寐欠佳，临厕努挣乏力，便质软。舌淡红，苔白厚（图 29）。脉细。

History of present illness: The patient gave birth thirty-one days ago. One weak ago, she began to fear wind. She reported heavy sensation in the body, lassitude, reduced appetite, restless sleep, and difficulty passing soft stool. Her tongue is reddish with white, thick coating (Fig. 29). Her pulse is thready.

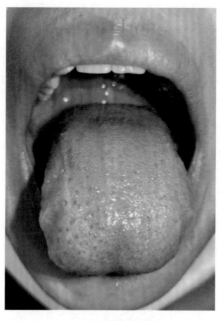

图 29　乓产呱（阴证）

Fig. 29　"Pingchangua" (yin syndrome)

目诊：白睛脉络浅淡。甲诊：甲色淡。壮医诊断：乒产呱（阴证）。中医诊断：产后病。西医诊断：产褥期疾病。

Eye examination: The blood vessels of the white of the eyes are reddish.

Nail examination: The nails are pale.

Diagnosis in ZM: "Pingchangua" characterized by yin syndrome.

Diagnosis in TCM: Puerperal diseases.

Diagnosis in WM: Postpartum diseases.

治疗原则：补虚，除瘀毒，祛风毒。

Treatment principles: Reinforce deficiency, and remove blood stasis and dispel wind.

治疗：壮医药浴疗法。

Treatment method: The ZM medicated bath therapy.

处方：黄花倒水莲 50 g，牛大力 50 g，五指毛桃 50 g，益母草 50 g，鸡屎藤 30 g，艾叶 20 g，路路通 20 g，防风 20 g，走马胎 20 g，生姜 30 g。

Prescription: Huanghuadaoshuilian (Radix seu Folium Polygalae Fallacis) 50 g, Niudali (Radix Millettiae Speciosae) 50 g, Wuzhimaotao (Radix Fici Hirtae) 50 g, Yimucao (Herba Leonuri) 50 g, Jishiteng (Herba Paederiae) 30 g, Aiye (Folium Artemisiae Argyi) 20 g, Lulutong (Fructus Liquidambaris) 20 g, Fangfeng (Radix Saposhnikoviae) 20 g, Zoumatai (Radix et Rhizoma Ardisiae Gigantifoliae) 20 g and Shengjiang (Rhizoma Zingiberis Recens) 30 g.

二诊（2020 年 5 月 22 日）：经壮医药浴疗法治疗 3 次后，畏风、身重乏力感明显缓解，二便正常，睡眠、饮食均佳。

Second visit (on May 22, 2020): After the patient took the ZM medicated bath three times, the symptom of intolerance of wind, heavy sensation in the body and lassitude had been relieved. She reported normal urination frequency, regular bowel movements, restful sleep and good appetite.

按语：本案患者产褥期出现畏风症状，自觉身重乏力，纳寐欠佳，临厕努挣乏力，便质软。舌淡红，苔白厚，脉细，属阴证。产后津血损伤，龙路空虚，元气受损。畏风、身重乏力均为龙路亏虚之象，谷道虚损不足可致临厕努挣但便质软，湿毒内生可见苔白厚。治宜以通调龙路、火路，补虚损，除湿毒为主。

采用壮医药浴疗法治疗，方中使用黄花倒水莲、牛大力、五指毛桃、益母草通龙路，补虚损，鸡屎藤、走马胎强筋骨，艾叶、路路通、防风、生姜除湿毒。诸药通过药浴合用，可使道路畅通，气血滋生，三气同步，畏风自除。

Summary statement: The patient reported intolerance of wind, heavy sensation in the body, reduced appetite, restless sleep, difficulty passing soft stool in her postpartum period. Her tongue was reddish with white, thick coating. Her pulse was thready. These manifestations signified yin syndrome. After childbirth, body fluid and blood are excessively consumed, leading to the emptiness of the dragon channel and deficiency of the original qi. Intolerance of wind, heavy sensation in the body and lassitude were the signs of the emptiness in the dragon channel. Consumption of the grain passage led to difficulty passing soft stool. The white, thick coating was the sign of interior dampness. Therefore, it was applicable to focus on regulating the dragon and fire channels, reducing consumption and removing dampness. In terms of the herbal medicinals used in the ZM medicated bath therapy, Huanghuadaoshuilian (Radix seu Folium Polygalae Fallacis), Niudali (Radix Millettiae Speciosae), Wuzhimaotao (Radix Fici Hirtae) and Yimucao (Herba Leonuri) were used to unblock the dragon channel and reduce consumption; Jishiteng (Herba Paederiae) and Zoumatai (Radix et Rhizoma Ardisiae Gigantifoliae) were used to strengthen tendons and bones; Aiye (Folium Artemisiae Argyi), Lulutong (Fructus Liquidambaris), Fangfeng (Radix Saposhnikoviae) and Shengjiang (Rhizoma Zingiberis Recens) were used to remove dampness. All these medicinals combined took the synergistic effect to unblock the two channels, nourish blood and qi and make the heaven-qi, earth-qi and human-qi synchronized. Consequently, the symptom of intolerance of wind vanished.

【病案三】

［Case 3］

钟某，女，40 岁，2020 年 6 月 11 日初诊。

Patient: Zhong, a 40-year-old woman, her first visit was on June 11, 2020.

主诉：产后易汗出 1 月余。

Chief complaint:"I have been liable to sweating after childbirth for more than one month."

现病史：1个多月前产后开始易出汗，动辄汗出，以冷汗为主，伴心悸，少气懒言，睡眠差，易怒，易上火，自产褥期至今一直未缓解，关脉细涩，寸浮。舌瘦暗，苔白（图30）。

History of present illness: The patient reported liability to sweating, which occurred more than one month ago. Sweating could be caused by light exertion and was marked by cold sweats. Accompanied symptoms include shortness of breath without desire to speak, restless sleep, irritability, and heatiness. All these symptoms had appeared at the beginning of the postpartum period, and had not been relieved until she came to seek medical care. Her Guan pulse is thready and unsmooth, and Cun pulse is floating. Her tongue is thin, dark red with white coating (Fig. 30).

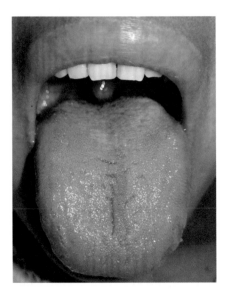

图 30　乒产呱（阴证）
Fig. 30　"Pingchangua" (yin syndrome)

目诊：白睛脉络12点钟方向色深红，曲张明显。甲诊：甲色红。壮医诊断：乒产呱（阴证）。中医诊断：产后病。西医诊断：产褥期疾病。

Eye examination: The blood vessels at the 12 o'clock position of the white of the eyes are dark red and apparently enlarged and twisted.

Nail examination: The nails are red.

Diagnosis in ZM:"Pingchangua" characterized by yin syndrome.

Diagnosis in TCM: Puerperal diseases.

Diagnosis in WM: Postpartum diseases.

治疗原则：补虚，除瘀毒，散寒毒，除湿毒。

Treatment principles: Reinforce deficiency, remove blood stasis, dispel cold and remove dampness.

治疗：壮医药浴疗法。

Treatment method: The ZM medicated bath therapy.

处方：黄花倒水莲 50 g，牛大力 50 g，扶芳藤 50 g，红花 20 g，牛膝 20 g，苏木 20 g，伸筋草 20 g，路路通 20 g，生姜 50 g，走马胎 30 g，艾叶 30 g。

Prescription: Huanghuadaoshuilian (Radix seu Folium Polygalae Fallacis) 50 g, Niudali (Radix Millettiae Speciosae) 50 g, Fufangteng (Caulis Euonymi Fortunei cum Foliis) 50 g, Honghua (Flos Carthami) 20 g, Niuxi (Radix Achyranthis Bidentatae) 20 g, Sumu (Lignum Sappan) 20 g, Shenjincao (Herba Lycopodii) 20 g, Lulutong (Fructus Liquidambaris) 20 g, Shengjiang (Rhizoma Zingiberis Recens) 50 g, Zoumatai (Radix et Rhizoma Ardisiae Gigantifoliae) 30 g and Aiye (Folium Artemisiae Argyi) 30 g.

使用方法：将药材煎煮成药液后，予全身药浴，每泡浴 5 分钟后坐起 2 分钟，如此循环 3 ～ 5 次。

Medicated bath method: Boil the herbal medicinals with water and pour the decoction into a large barrel. Leave the whole body to soak in the barrel for 5 minutes and then sit up in it for 2 minutes, which is repeated 3 to 5 times.

二诊（2020 年 8 月 13 日）：经壮医药浴疗法治疗 10 次后，易出汗明显缓解，二便正常，睡眠、饮食好转。

Second visit (on August 13, 2020): After the patient took the ZM medicated bath ten times, liability to sweating had been significantly relieved. She reported normal urination frequency, regular bowel movements, better sleep and appetite.

按语：本案患者就诊时一直可见易出汗，动辄汗出，以冷汗为主，伴心悸，少气懒言，睡眠差，易怒，易上火，自产褥期至今一直未缓解，舌瘦暗，苔白，寸浮，关脉细涩，属阴证。产时耗气伤血，脉络空虚，在复原过程中，瘀血易停、滞留，寒毒易乘机外犯直入。易汗出、心悸、少气懒言均为龙路空虚所致，冷汗提示兼挟寒邪，火路不通可致睡眠差，易怒，易上火。治宜以通调龙路、火路，补虚损，除寒毒为主。黄花倒水莲、牛大力、扶芳藤通调龙路、火路，补虚损，走马胎强筋骨，红花、牛膝散瘀毒，苏木、伸筋草、路路通通经络，艾叶、生姜散寒毒。诸药通过药浴合用，可使道路畅通，气血滋生，三气同步，易汗出自除。

Summary statement: The patient reported liability to sweating which lasted from the beginning of her postpartum period until she sought medical care. The sweating could be caused by light exertion and was marked by cold sweats. Accompanied symptoms included shortness of breath without desire to speak, restless sleep, irritability and heatiness. Her tongue was thin and dark red with white coating. Her Cun pulse was floating and Guan pulse was thready and unsmooth. These manifestations signified yin syndrome. Excessive consumption of qi and blood during delivery leads to meridian emptiness. During recovery, static blood tends to stagnate. As a result, cold is more likely to invade the body. Excessive sweating, palpitation, shortness of breath and without desire to speak were caused by the emptiness of the dragon channel. Cold sweats meant pathogenic cold. The obstruction of the fire channel led to restless sleep, irritability and heatiness. Therefore, it was applicable to regulate these two channels, reduce consumption and remove cold. In terms of the herbal medicinals used in the ZM medicated bath therapy, Huanghuadaoshuilian (Radix seu Folium Polygalae Fallacis), Niudali (Radix Millettiae Speciosae) and Fufangteng (Caulis Euonymi Fortunei cum Foliis) were used to reduce consumption; Zoumatai (Radix et Rhizoma Ardisiae Gigantifoliae) was used to strengthen tendons and bones; Honghua (Flos Carthami) and Niuxi (Radix Achyranthis Bidentatae) were used to remove blood stasis; Sumu (Lignum Sappan), Shenjincao (Herba Lycopodii) and Lulutong (Fructus Liquidambaris) were used to unblock the meridians and collaterals; and Aiye (Folium Artemisiae Argyi) and Shengjiang (Rhizoma Zingiberis Recens) were used to remove cold. All the herbal medicinals combined took synergistic effect to unblock the two channels, nourish blood and qi and make the heaven-qi, earth-qi and human-qi synchronized. Consequently, the symptom of liability to sweating vanished.